Nephrology

Editor

SAMUEL SNYDER

PRIMARY CARE: CLINICS IN OFFICE PRACTICE

www.primarycare.theclinics.com

Consulting Editor
JOEL J. HEIDELBAUGH

December 2014 • Volume 41 • Number 4

ELSEVIER

1600 John F. Kennedy Boulevard • Suite 1800 • Philadelphia, Pennsylvania, 19103-2899

http://www.theclinics.com

PRIMARY CARE: CLINICS IN OFFICE PRACTICE Volume 41, Number 4
December 2014 ISSN 0095-4543, ISBN-13: 978-0-323-32674-2

Editor: Jessica McCool
Developmental Editor: Yonah Korngold

Primary Care: Clinics in Office Practice (ISSN: 0095–4543) is published quarterly by Elsevier Inc., 360 Park Avenue South, New York, NY 10010-1710. Months of issue are March, June, September, and December. Periodicals postage paid at New York, NY and additional mailing offices. Subscription prices are $225.00 per year (US individuals), $392.00 (US institutions), $115.00 (US students), $275.00 (Canadian individuals), $444.00 (Canadian institutions), $175.00 (Canadian students), $345.00 (international individuals), $444.00 (international institutions), and $175.00 (international students). Foreign air speed delivery is included in all *Clinics* subscription prices. All prices are subject to change without notice. POSTMASTER: Send address changes to *Primary Care: Clinics in Office Practice*, Elsevier Periodicals Customer Service, 11830 Westline Industrial Drive, St. Louis, MO 63146. Customer Service Health Sciences Division, Subscription Customer Service, 3251 Riverport Lane, Maryland Heights, MO 63043. **Customer Service: 1-800-654-2452 (U.S. and Canada); 314-447-8871 (outside U.S. and Canada). Fax: 314-447-8029. E-mail: journalscustomerservice-usa@elsevier.com (for print support); journalsonlinesupport-usa@elsevier.com (for online support).**

Reprints. For copies of 100 or more, of articles in this publication, please contact the Commercial Reprints Department, Elsevier Inc., 360 Park Avenue South, New York, NY 10010-1710. Tel. 212-633-3874; Fax: 212-633-3820; E-mail: reprints@elsevier.com.

Primary Care: Clinics in Office Practice is covered in *MEDLINE/PubMed (Index Medicus)* and *EMBASE/Excerpta Medica, Current Contents/Clinical Medicine,* and *ISI/BIOMED.*

Contributors

CONSULTING EDITOR

JOEL J. HEIDELBAUGH, MD, FAAFP, FACG
Clinical Professor, Departments of Family Medicine and Urology; Clerkship Director, Department of Family Medicine, University of Michigan Medical School, Ann Arbor, Michigan; Ypsilanti Health Center, Ypsilanti, Michigan

EDITOR

SAMUEL SNYDER, DO, FACP, FACOI, FASN
Professor and Chair, Department of Internal Medicine, Nova Southeastern University College of Osteopathic Medicine, Fort Lauderdale, Florida; and Program Director, Osteopathic Internal Medicine Residency, Mount Sinai Medical Center, Miami Beach, Florida

AUTHORS

GHULAM AKBAR, MD
Division of Nephrology, Department of Medicine, Lankenau Medical Center, Wynnewood, Pennsylvania

MARK D. BALDWIN, DO, FACOI
Assistant Clinical Professor of Medicine, Ohio University of Osteopathic Medicine, Athens, Ohio; Private Practice, Columbus, Ohio

ROBERT L. BENZ, MD, FACP
Chief, Division of Nephrology, Main Line Health System, Lankenau Medical Center; Professor of Medicine, Thomas Jefferson University Medical Center, Lankenau Nephrology Fellowship Program Director and Vice President of Medical Affairs, Lankenau Institute of Medical Research, Wynnewood, Pennsylvania

JASON BIEDERMAN, DO, FACOI, FASN
Garden City Hospital, Garden City, Michigan; Hypertension Nephrology Associates, PC, Livonia, Michigan

PARHAM EFTEKHARI, DO, MSc
Clinical Assistant Professor of Medicine, Broward Health Medical Center, Nova Southeastern University College of Osteopathic Medicine, Fort Lauderdale, Florida

ELIZABETH HAMES, DO
Assistant Professor, Department of Geriatrics, Nova Southeastern University College of Osteopathic Medicine; Assistant Program Director, Geriatric Medicine Fellowship, Broward Health Medical Center, Nova Southeastern University, Fort Lauderdale, Florida

JONES SAM JOHN, DO
Nephrology Fellow, Nephrology Department, Allegheny General Hospital, Pittsburgh, Pennsylvania

SAIFULLAH N. KAZI, MBBS, MD
Nephrology Fellow, Lankenau Medical Center and Research Institute, Wynnewood, Pennsylvania

ANTHONY MALCOUN, DO
Director, Nephrology Fellowship Program, St John Health System, Warren, Michigan; Hypertension Nephrology Associate, PC, Livonia, Michigan; Clinical Professor of Medicine, Michigan State College of Osteopathic Medicine East Lansing, Michigan; Division of Nephrology, St. John Macomb Hospital, Warren, Michigan

HADY MASRI, DO
Assistant Professor, Department of Geriatrics, Nova Southeastern University College of Osteopathic Medicine; Interim Program Director, Geriatric Medicine Fellowship, Broward Health Medical Center, Nova Southeastern University, Fort Lauderdale, Florida

KELLY MERCIER, DO
Botsford Hospital, Farmington Hills, Michigan

FERNANDO PEDRAZA, MD
Division of Nephrology and Hypertension, University of Miami Miller School of Medicine, Miami, Florida

RAGHAVESH PULLALAREVU, MD
Division of Nephrology, Department of Medicine, Lankenau Medical Center, Wynnewood, Pennsylvania

SAADUR RAHMAN, DO
Nephrology Fellow, Garden City Hospital, Michigan State University, Garden City, Michigan

KENYA M. RIVAS VELASQUEZ, MD
Assistant Professor and Vice Chair, Department of Geriatrics, Nova Southeastern University College of Osteopathic Medicine, Fort Lauderdale-Davie, Florida

DAVID ROTH, MD
Division of Nephrology and Hypertension, Miami Transplant Institute, University of Miami Miller School of Medicine, Miami, Florida

HOLLY SMITH, DO
Garden City Hospital, Garden City, Michigan

SAMUEL SNYDER, DO, FACP, FACOI, FASN
Professor and Chair, Department of Internal Medicine, Nova Southeastern University College of Osteopathic Medicine, Fort Lauderdale, Florida; and Program Director, Osteopathic Internal Medicine Residency, Mount Sinai Medical Center, Miami Beach, Florida

GEOFFREY TEEHAN, MD, MS, FACP
Division of Nephrology, Department of Medicine, Lankenau Institute of Medical Research, Lankenau Medical Center, Wynnewood, Pennsylvania

ALAN TURNER, DO
Resident, Internal Medicine at Mount Sinai Medical Center, Miami Beach, Florida

GRACIE A. TURNER, DO, MPH
Chief Resident, Internal Medicine at Mount Sinai Medical Center, Miami Beach, Florida

JACK WATERMAN, DO, FACOI
Clinical Associate Professor of Medicine, Nova Southeastern University College of Osteopathic Medicine, Fort Lauderdale, Florida; Medical Director, Jupiter Kidney Center, Jupiter, Florida

Contents

Angiotensin-converting enzyme (ACE) inhibitor or angiotensin receptor blocker (ARB) therapy in hypertensive diabetic patients with macroalbuminuria, microalbuminuria, or normoalbuminuria has been repeatedly shown to improve cardiovascular mortality and reduce the decline in glomerular filtration rate. Renin-angiotensin-aldosterone system (RAAS) blockade in normotensive diabetic patients with normoalbuminuria or microalbuminuria cannot be advocated at present. Dual RAAS inhibition with ACE inhibitors plus ARBs or ACE inhibitors plus direct renin inhibitors has failed to improve cardiovascular or renal outcomes but has predisposed patients to serious adverse events.

Acute kidney injury (AKI) is becoming more prevalent in the hospital setting and is associated with the worst prognostic outcomes, including increased mortality. Many different factors contribute to the development of AKI in hospitalized patients, including medications, older age, sepsis, and comorbid conditions. Correct evaluation and management of AKI requires investigation and understanding of important causative factors for each of the 3 pathophysiologic categories of renal failure. Preventative efforts rely on prompt recognition of AKI while avoiding iatrogenic insults in the hospital setting.

Nonsteroidal antiinflammatory drugs (NSAIDs) are one of the most commonly used classes of medications in the world, which function by inhibiting the cyclooxygenase (COX) enzymes and downregulating the inflammatory pathway. COX enzymes are constitutively expressed in the kidneys and function to maintain a homeostatic environment in terms of maintaining the glomerular filtration rate, blood pressure, sodium, water, and osmotic regulation. When the COX enzymes are inhibited by NSAIDs, a multitude of renal and vascular complications occur. This article aims to enlighten primary care physicians of the complications that arise with NSAIDs from a renal perspective and to present some management strategies.

Renal cysts are commonly encountered in clinical practice. Although most cysts found on routine imaging studies are benign, there must be an index of suspicion to exclude a neoplastic process or the presence of a multicystic disorder. This article focuses on the more common adult cystic diseases, including simple and complex renal cysts, autosomal-dominant polycystic kidney disease, and acquired cystic kidney disease.

Chronic kidney disease (CKD) continues to be an ever-increasing health problem in the United States and elsewhere. Diabetes mellitus and hypertension remain the primary causes, and much of this is related to increased rates of obesity. Studies have demonstrated that early referral to a nephrologist can be life-saving and can also markedly improve quality of life. Besides recommending treatments for CKD, early referral can assist in medication management and in minimizing exposure to potential nephrotoxins. In patients who progress to end-stage renal disease, having an established patient-PCP-nephrologist relationship can ease the transition to renal replacement therapy or transplantation.

Chronic kidney disease (CKD) has a high prevalence in the elderly population. Almost half of the population reaches moderate impairment (CKD 3) by 65 years of age. This article describes CKD staging in the geriatric population and several common clinical presentations of renal disease. Diagnosis and treatment regimens of CKD are discussed. Geriatric patients are at an increased risk for renal dysfunction from many causes. Some causes are inherent with aging, such as gross structural and cellular changes, decrease in physiologic function, and lowered vascular compensatory reserve. Exposures, including medications and diagnostic testing, are contributors to acute kidney injury.

The prevalence of chronic kidney disease (CKD) is increasing, and the epidemic of obesity is one of the causes. Obesity exacerbates hypertension as a risk factor for CKD, causing vasoconstriction and salt and water retention. Obesity also worsens glucose intolerance and insulin resistance as risk factors for CKD. Obesity targets the kidney by triggering novel pathways of intrarenal inflammation, recruiting professional immunologic cells through metaflammation. Obesity-related glomerulopathy has emerged as a distinct pathologic variant of focal segmental glomerulosclerosis. No definitive treatments have come about for obesity-related glomerulopathy, but among the most promising prospects is aggressive weight loss, including bariatric surgery.

Kidney transplant recipients (KTRs) commonly present with complex medical issues that are best managed jointly by both their primary care physician and the kidney transplant center. Hypertension, diabetes, dyslipidemias, and obesity are frequently present in the KTR population and the successful management of these comorbidities is essential in achieving excellent posttransplant outcomes. Cardiovascular disease is the leading cause of mortality in KTRs, and interventions that mitigate the risk factors that contribute to these adverse outcomes are an important part of the long-term management of a KTR.

PRIMARY CARE:
CLINICS IN OFFICE PRACTICE

Foreword

"I Don't Take Creatinine"

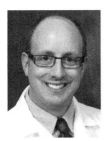

Joel J. Heidelbaugh, MD, FAAFP, FACG
Consulting Editor

With the incorporation of the Affordable Care Act, many of us are seeing dozens of new patients entering our practices. Last week, I saw a young and very muscular man for a health maintenance exam, which was his first doctor's visit in over 8 years, because he said that he "had always been healthy." I immediately noticed that his blood pressure was 161/96 and obtained a routine panel of blood tests that revealed a serum creatinine of 1.9 mg/dL and an estimated glomerular filtration rate of 49 mL/min. I asked my nurses to arrange for a follow-up visit to recheck his blood pressure and discuss the results of his blood tests; his repeat blood pressure 3 days later was 165/90. It was a pleasure for me to have this patient establish care with my practice since, if he hadn't found a doctor, he would have continued to have undiagnosed and untreated hypertension and stage 3 chronic kidney disease (CKD).

In further evaluation, I also discovered that he has prediabetes, hyperlipidemia, and nephrotic-range proteinuria. During the follow-up visit, I took the opportunity to explain to the patient some basic pathophysiology of the kidney as well as the significance of his lab results. After a few minutes of what I thought was relatively simple analogies to explain complex medical terms he replied, "I don't take creatinine; I'm naturally strong, so there must be a mistake."

A recent study published in the *New England Journal of Medicine* determined that acute kidney injury (AKI) and CKD are likely to be interconnected, suggesting that patients who develop one condition are likely to develop the other at some point, augmenting the need for clinicians to be hypervigilant in their patients, especially those with chronic diseases including diabetes mellitus.[1] This issue of *Primary Care: Clinics in Office Practice* provides detailed summaries of the current literature on subtopics germane to the principles and practices of nephrology. The articles are dedicated to common renal conditions, including proteinuria, hematuria, renal cysts, AKI, and CKD. A review of the relationship between obesity and the development of kidney disease provides insight into a potentially controllable relationship. As we continue to encounter greater numbers of patients with CKD, the need for primary care clinicians

Prim Care Clin Office Pract 41 (2014) xi–xii
http://dx.doi.org/10.1016/j.pop.2014.10.001
0095-4543/14/$ – see front matter © 2014 Elsevier Inc. All rights reserved.
primarycare.theclinics.com

to interact with nephrologists and comanage their patients will certainly grow more imperative.

Nephrology is amazingly complicated. We lack curative therapies to reverse and cure most diseases of the kidney, and the need for dialysis will increase in the coming decades. As the rates of kidney disease rise and the population ages, the need for research and skilled clinicians will become substantially greater. In the 2014 Fellowship Match, only 91 US internal medicine residents applied for a nephrology fellowship, with only 76% of available positions filling with both US and foreign medical school graduates.[2] The only internal medicine subspecialty field to match fewer total residents was geriatrics.[2] These statistics prove that the impending shortage in nephrologists will place a great demand on primary care clinicians to diagnose and manage many diseases of the kidney, as well as manage those patients with end-stage kidney disease who are on dialysis.

I offer my gratitude to Dr Samuel Snyder and his colleagues for their efforts in the arduous task of developing an issue of articles on renal diseases to serve as a reference for primary care clinicians, as it is quite a remarkable and thorough compendium. While prevention of most kidney diseases is not possible, with the solid foundation of knowledge that lies herein, it is hoped that we can detect more cases of kidney disease early on and provide appropriate treatment and coordination of care with our nephrology colleagues.

Joel J. Heidelbaugh, MD, FAAFP, FACG
Departments of Family Medicine and Urology
University of Michigan Medical School
Ann Arbor, MI 48109, USA

Ypsilanti Health Center
200 Arnet Street, Suite 200
Ypsilanti, MI 48198, USA

E-mail address:
jheidel@umich.edu

REFERENCES

1. Chalwa LS, Eggers PW, Star RA, et al. Acute kidney injury and chronic kidney disease as interconnected syndromes. New Engl J Med 2014;371(1):58–66.
2. Results and Data—Specialties Matching Service. The Match—National Resident Matching Program. 2014 Appointment Year. Available at: www.nrmp.org/wp-content/uploads/2013/08/National-Resident-Matching-Program-NRMP-Results-and-Data-SMS-2014-Final.pdf. Accessed September 20, 2014.

Preface

Ambulatory Nephrology

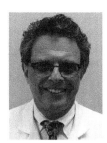

Samuel Snyder, DO, FACP, FACOI, FASN
Editor

You can't do it all in one small issue.

There is a rising tide of kidney disease in the United States. The major causes continue to be diabetes and hypertension, and now, the impact of obesity magnifies the effect of these. It is difficult to ascertain the prevalence of chronic kidney disease (CKD) with precision, but we know this much. From 1973 when Medicare established the End Stage Renal Disease program, ESRD has grown from 10,000 patients to over 615,000 patients in 2012.[1] Based on extrapolation from NHANES III data, using decreased eGFR as the defining criterion (stage 3 or higher CKD), the prevalence of CKD in the United States might be as high as 10.4%.[2] Consideration of proteinuria improves the predictive power of eGFR for predicting risk of progression of kidney disease.[3] The impact of this tide is that CKD is associated with greater risks of cardiovascular morbidity and mortality, and in fact, all cause mortality, as well as greater consumption of health care resources.[4,5] Hence, there is a need for greater understanding and more aggressive investigation and treatment.

The range of problems to which the kidney is heir is deep and wide. The signs and symptoms of kidney disease are final common pathways through which many insults are expressed. Often these expressions surface first in the primary care physician's office. As the prevalence of kidney disease is increasing, its diagnosis and initial management are falling more commonly to the primary care physician. It is our goal here to update the primary care physician about several classic presentations and to present a sample of the some current problems in nephrology as they impact primary care.

Classic problems include proteinuria, hematuria, and renal cysts. We present contemporary perspectives on these problems to streamline the diagnostic approach according to current understanding.

The most prevalent disease in the United States is hypertension. The percentage of hypertension that is secondary rather than essential is considered to be increasing. We present a review of secondary hypertension, covering the appropriate indices of suspicion, and workup. In addition, we present a state-of-the-art review on the use of

http://dx.doi.org/10.1016/j.pop.2014.09.002
0095-4543/14/$

angiotensin-converting-enzyme inhibitors and receptor blockers in the use of hypertension, heart disease, and kidney disease.

Acute kidney injury is presented in two aspects. One of the most widely prescribed drug classes—and widely used over the counter—is nonsteroidal anti-inflammatory drugs, including COX2s. We present a current review of this subject, which remains timely despite our long experience with this serious and common problem. The single article in this collection that is not based mostly in outpatient medicine is the article on nosocomial acute kidney injury. However, the focus is still on primary care, and the emphasis is on prevention of this complication of modern medicine.

Because of the increasing prevalence of chronic kidney disease, its management is increasingly a problem in which the primary care physician and the nephrologist must act cooperatively on behalf of our patients. We present several aspects of the spectrum of CKD, including a perspective on how the partnership between nephrologist and primary care physician might look as the patient progresses through the stages of CKD. As our population ages, the prevalence of CKD in the geriatric population increases, and the special needs of this growing subset are considered. Of course, the optimal treatment for end-stage CKD is transplant, and the kidney transplant patient presents more frequently than ever before to the office of his primary care physician, so this is a group that requires special consideration as well. This issue also presents a state-of-the-art review of the fastest-growing epidemic in America: the epidemic of obesity. In order to increase awareness of this problem, this article discusses how the epidemic of obesity targets the kidney as well as the heart and is a growing cause of CKD.

It is impossible to be comprehensive about the practice of ambulatory nephrology in any single issue. But it is our hope to present a useful collection of the more common challenges in nephrology with which the primary care physician must be familiar and to stimulate your interest in further reading.

Samuel Snyder, DO, FACP, FACOI, FASN
Nova Southeastern University College of Osteopathic Medicine
Fort Lauderdale, FL, USA

Osteopathic Internal Medicine Residency
Mt. Sinai Medical Center
Miami Beach, FL, USA

E-mail address:
snyderdo@nova.edu

REFERENCES

1. United States Renal Data System. USRDS 2013 Annual Data Report: Atlas of Chronic Kidney Disease and End Stage Renal Disease in the United States. Bethesda (MD): National Institutes of Health, National Institute of Diabetes and Digestive and Kidney Diseases; 2013.
2. Coresh J, Selvin E, Stevens LA, et al. Prevalence of chronic kidney disease in the United States. JAMA 2007;298:2038–47.
3. Hallan SI, Ritz E, Lydersen S, et al. Combining GFR and albuminuria to classify CKD improves prediction of ESRD. J Am Soc Nephrol 2009;20:1069–77.
4. Go AS, Chertow GM, Fan D, et al. Chronic kidney disease and the risks of death, cardiovascular events and hospitalization. N Engl J Med 2004;351:1296–305.
5. Khan SS, Kasmi WH, Abichandani R, et al. Health care utilization among patients with chronic kidney disease. Kidney Int 2002;62:229–36.

Workup for Proteinuria

Samuel Snyder, DO[a], Jones Sam John, DO[b],*

KEYWORDS

- Proteinuria • Glomerulus in the prevention of proteinuria • Proteinuria workup
- Complications with proteinuria • General treatments in patient with proteinuria

KEY POINTS

- The history, physical, and initial laboratory workup, including urinalysis with microscopy, is key to determining the etiology chronic kidney disease.
- Proteinuria is an early sign of renal disease.
- Proteinuria is associated with microvascular complications and mortality, which must be anticipated and prevented.

INTRODUCTION

The kidney is fundamentally a filter that has numerous elegant properties and filtration characteristics. Like all filters, it is supposed to let some things through (waste products) and keep other things from going through (large proteins and essential elements). Disturbances in this filter manifest as proteinuria. Although some benign conditions present with proteinuria, proteinuria is generally a marker for renal disease, a manifestation of systemic disease in the kidney, a risk factor for kidney disease progression, or a marker for cardiovascular disease.[1-3] Chronic kidney disease (CKD) evaluation guidelines from the Kidney Disease Initiative Global Outcomes (KDIGO) changed in 2012 to include the degree of proteinuria to classify CKD, in addition to the estimated glomerular filtration rate (eGFR).[4] Although the leading causes of CKD leading to end-stage renal disease (ESRD) requiring dialysis in the United States are diabetes and hypertension,[5] it is important to know how to initiate a workup for other causes of renal dysfunction as well, because early referral to a nephrologist has shown to prevent further renal damage and mortality.[6-8] In this article, we discuss glomerular structure, definition of proteinuria, general workup for proteinuria from a primary care standpoint, classification of diseases, the significance and complications of proteinuria, and general aspects of treatment.

Disclosures: None.
[a] 3200 South University Drive, Fort Lauderdale, FL 33328, USA; [b] Nephrology Department, Allegheny General Hospital, 4th Floor, 320 East North Avenue, Pittsburgh, PA 15212, USA
* Corresponding author.
E-mail address: jjohn@wpahs.org

HOW PROTEINURIA OCCURS: GLOMERULAR STRUCTURE AND FUNCTION

The kidney normally prevents most protein from reaching the final urine. Plasma reaches the glomerulus of Bowman's capsule at the rate of 180 L/d and is filtered across the glomerular basement membrane (GBM). This unique filtration mechanism is accomplished by a complex mix of glycoproteins, sialoproteins, and type 4A collagen with multiple subunits, which extrudes from the mesangial cells supporting the tuft of glomerular capillaries, and layered over the capillary loops in 3 layers: The lamina rara interna, lamina dura, and lamina rara externa (**Fig. 1**). The molecular size, steric features, and electric charge of the compounds in plasma, along with GBM's sieving characteristics, determine filtration. The space between endothelial cells on the capillary lumen form fenestrae (Latin for *windows*), which are the initial portals for filtration through which plasma transits, based on the transcapillary pressure gradient. Plasma then meets the lamina rara interna, which has collagen IV $\alpha3\alpha4\alpha5$ (missing in Alport's syndrome), which provides strength against the filtration forces.[9] This layer has negatively charged glycosaminoglycans, which provide an electrostatic barrier against negatively charged proteins (especially albumin), preventing passage. Plasma then passes through the lamina dura, which contains both type 4A collagen as well as laminin, and acts as a selective filter for macromolecules. Before entering Bowmans' space, plasma passes through the lamina rara externa adjacent to podocytes, the foot processes of epithelial cells in Bowman's space. Podocytes normally bear a negative charge along their external surface, thus repelling negatively charged particles in plasma filtrate. This negative charge also repels the walls of adjacent podocytes, which accounts for the typical appearance of separate foot processes.[10,11] Podocytes are attached to the GBM with stabilizing proteins such as actin, and produce proteins that regulate motility and interaction between cells and matrix.[12] The sieving coefficient of the GBM does not normally allow molecules as large or as negatively charged as albumin ($\sim$67 kD) to pass through into the Bowman's space. Thus, there should be little or no albumin present in the final urine (<30 mg/dL/d). Thus, if albumin is present, it is a clear indicator of glomerular damage.

Once plasma filtrate is in Bowman's capsule, it proceeds down the proximal convoluted tubule. Although most albumin, immunoglobulins, and other large molecular weight proteins have been rejected by the GBM, the filtrate would contain small

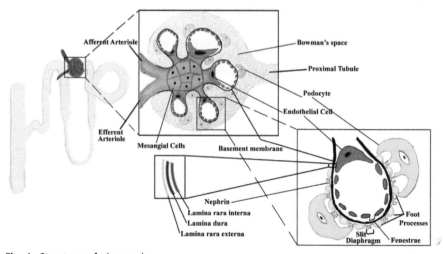

Fig. 1. Structure of glomerulus.

molecular weight proteins and peptides that are positively charged. As these molecules reach the brush border of the proximal tubular epithelial cells, they are reabsorbed from the filtrate by epithelial transport mechanisms or endocytosis, catabolized, and their components returned to the systemic circulation.[11]

Further down the nephron, epithelial cells of the ascending loop of Henle secrete the glycoprotein uromodulin, previously called Tamm Horsfall protein. As a monomer, this protein is 68 kDa, but can accumulate in the urine in aggregates of more than 1 million Dalton. This protein is usually in liquid state in the urine. However, in conditions of low flow or alkaline pH, it may precipitate in a gel form. It forms the matrix of casts and may also be a part of the matrix of stones. It can appear in urine in significant quantities in benign conditions or in the company of immunoglobulins. Even though the function of uromodulin is not fully understood, there is some suggestion that it protects against urinary tract infections and kidney stone formation, and it may also be seen in larger quantities in the urine of individuals with CKD and hypertension.[13]

IDENTIFICATION AND QUANTIFICATION OF PROTEINURIA

Urine dipsticks are often the first indication of proteinuria in the office. The dipstick is both qualitative and semiquantitative. The degree of proteinuria encountered on a urine dipstick must be interpreted in the light of the concentration of the urine determined by the specific gravity of the urine. Thus, a ++ reading in a well-hydrated patient producing large quantities of urine may signify a much greater quantity of protein than a ++ reading in a dehydrated patient producing only small amounts protein, because the concentration of the urine in the dehydrated patient would be higher. Dipsticks that show ++++ reading often signify greater than 1 g of protein per 24 hours, but there is no way to be certain by dipstick how much greater than 1 g of protein there may be.[14] The pad on most urine dipsticks that detects protein contains tetrabromophenol blue and citrate buffer; however, other dyes that are more specific and sensitive to albumin are also available.[15,16] The electronegativity of proteins causes the dye on the pad to change colors from yellow to blue. Proteins like immunoglobulins that have a positive charge do not change the color of the indicator and thus lead to false-negative dipstick results. An increase in the alkalinity of the urine also causes the indicator to change color (**Table 1**).[16]

The dipstick is more or less selective for albuminuria, as discussed. Usually, sulfosalicylic acid (SSA) is used to detect proteins such as immunoglobulins. A few drops of SSA flocculate immunoglobulins in the urine. Thus, positive results of urine dipstick and SSA may prompt one to seek greater characterization of the types of protein present by ordering immunelectrophoresis or immunofixation of urine or blood, to look for paraproteinemias such as myeloma.

If one of the described tests is positive, then the proteinuria should be quantified promptly and accurately. The classic method of protein quantification is a 24-hour

Table 1		
False readings in urine dipstick and benign causes of proteinuria		
False Positive	**False Negative**	**Benign Causes of Proteinuria**
Dehydration	Overhydration	Fever
UTI	Positively charged proteins (light chains)	Acute illness
Hematuria		Exercise
Alkaline urine pH>8		Orthostatic proteinuria
Recent exercise		

urine collection. However, this process is fraught with error. Many times the specimen is overcollected (urine collected for >24 hours) or undercollected (urine collected for <24 hours), so proper collection must be explained carefully to the patient. Checking urine creatinine in the same 24-hour collection helps to ensure the accuracy of the collection. Creatinine excretion is proportional to muscle mass, which in turn varies with age and gender. Males generally excrete about 20 to 25 mg/kg/d and females excrete about 15 to 20 mg/kg/d. For example, a young or middle-aged 70-kg man should have about 1400 to 1850 mg of creatinine in a 24-hour collection. The amount of creatinine is expected to be lower in the elderly population owing to decreased muscle mass. Calculating this repeatedly to determine the accuracy of 24-hour collections can become cumbersome quickly.

Alternatively, proteinuria can be estimated by looking at the ratio of protein and creatinine in a spot urine specimen. The ratio is more accurate than urine dipstick and approximates the 24-hour protein excretion in grams per day fairly accurately.[14] Assuming an average person in a steady state excretes about 1 g of creatinine daily, the denominator of the ratio is 1. A 24-hour urine collection at some point in the patient's workup provides a true denominator for the ratio, and can be used throughout the course of the patient's care.

CLINICAL FINDINGS/CLASSIFICATION: HOW TO WORK UP THE PATIENT WITH PROTEINURIA

In nephrology, as in many other aspects of medicine, a thorough initial history is vital to determining the true etiology of a disease process. The underlying disease process may be discovered by kidney biopsy, and often biopsy is necessary to secure the diagnosis. However, the inciting factor needs to be determined to provide some idea about prognosis, prevent further injury, or prevent relapse of the disease in a transplanted kidney. In fact, the biopsy cannot stand alone, but must be interpreted in light of the patient's history and serologic findings. By thorough history collection (including family history, social history, and medication history) and workup for the suspected etiology, one can usually pinpoint a few causes of insult, and if needed, a kidney biopsy will help to make the diagnosis certain.

The first step is to determine whether the findings are benign based on history. For example, it is common to find a gram or less of urinary protein in the setting of fever, heart failure, seizures, or post exercise. So in that setting, a repeat dipstick should be performed in 4 to 6 weeks, unless there is interval change in symptoms, before a more extensive workup is undertaken.

There is daytime proteinuria in about 3% of the normal population younger than 30. Those individuals have no other significant findings suggested in the history, physical, or other laboratory workup. This is thought to be benign without any long-term decline in renal function. In this situation, a 24-hour split urine can be obtained (where the daytime urine is separated from an 8 hour nighttime urine sample). This split would show no protein in the nighttime collection, but the daytime collection would have protein, generally subnephrotic. This diagnosis can also be ruled out if early morning first void urine is negative for protein.

The kidney's function is not limited to waste clearance and recollection of vital organic compounds; it is also a vascular neuroendocrine organ that adapts to the needs of the body. As such, kidney disease can be thought of as either localized injury at the level of the kidney (primary/idiopathic) or as sequelae of a systemic insult/illness (secondary). It can be further categorized by the amount of protein found on quantification as nephrotic (>3.5 g/d) or nephritic range proteinuria (<3 g/d; **Table 2**). There is

Table 2
Degrees of proteinuria

Parameter	Category
Proteinuria (mg/d)	
<150	Normal
150–3000	Nephritic
>3500	Nephrotic
Albuminuria (mg/d)	
<30	Normal
30–300	Microalbuminuria
>300	Macroalbuminuria

a spectrum of presentations, and diseases that are generally thought to have nephritic range proteinuria may have nephrotic range proteinuria and vice versa. The diseases can also be categorized based on where in the kidney the damage is occurring. For instance, albuminuria represents glomerular disease, whereas nonalbumin protein may represent tubular disease, or in the case of immunoglobulins, primary hematologic disease.

The workup is based on disease history, or active disease present, and findings from serum chemistry (including blood urea nitrogen and creatinine), complete blood count, liver enzymes, lipid panel, serum albumin level, urinalysis with microscopy, and renal ultrasonography. Serologic studies can be ordered based on these findings and diagnostic probabilities.

Urine microscopy helps in determining the origin of the disease. Red blood cell (RBC) casts and dysmorphic RBCs indicate a glomerular pathology. Granular casts and tubular cells seen under the microscope might suggest acute tubular necrosis. Crystals may be seen on microscopy indicating crystal nephropathy. Maltese crosses are present under polarized light if there is lipid present, which indicates nephrotic range proteinuria and nephrotic syndrome. In those with nephrotic range proteinuria with history that is not suggestive of an etiology, serum protein electrophoresis, urine protein electrophoresis, urine immunofixation electrophoresis, and serum free light chains can be obtained to rule out myeloma.

Patients who have features suggestive of recent infection and now have renal manifestations, anti–streptolysin O antibodies, complement levels (low C3 and CH50 but normal C4), and streptozyme may be done in addition to blood cultures to diagnose post streptococcal glomerulonephritis.

In patients with pulmonary hemorrhage and renal manifestations (hematuria, RBC casts, dysmorphic RBCs), positive anti-GBM will give the diagnosis of Goodpasture disease.

Antineutrophil cytoplasm antibodies is positive in those with vasculitis, in particular granulomatosis polyangitis (formerly known as Wegner's granulomatosis) with c-antineutrophil cytoplasm antibodies and specificity of proteinase-3 and microscopic polyangitis with p-antineutrophil cytoplasm antibodies and specificity of myeloperoxidase. These vasculitides may present with rapidly declining renal function.

If history or presentation is suggestive of membranoproliferative glomerulonephritis, obtaining complement levels are helpful in distinguishing between membranoproliferative glomerulonephritis I (low C3 and C4) and membranoproliferative glomerulonephritis III (normal C4, but low C3; **Fig. 2**; **Table 3**).[17]

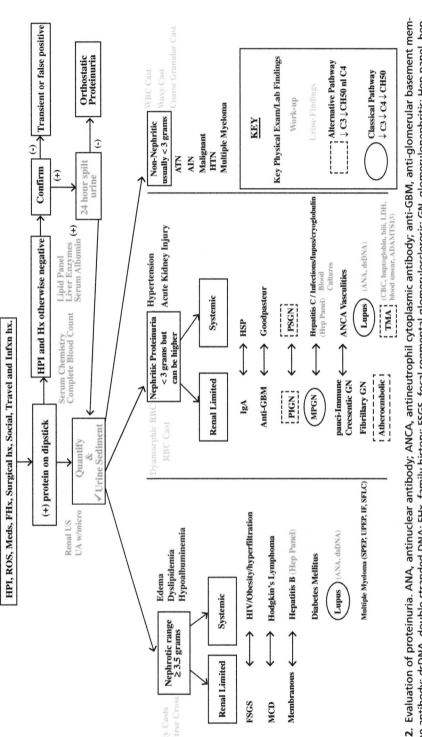

Fig. 2. Evaluation of proteinuria. ANA, antinuclear antibody; ANCA, antineutrophil cytoplasmic antibody; anti-GBM, anti-glomerular basement membrane antibody; dsDNA, double-stranded DNA; FHx, family history; FSGS, focal segmental glomerulosclerosis; GN, glomerulonephritis; Hep panel, hepatitis panel; HPI, history of present illness; HSP, Henoch–Schönlein purpura; Hx, history; IF, immunofixation; Infxn, infection; MCD, minimal change disease; MPGN, membranoproliferative glomerulonephritis; PIGN, postinfectious glomerulonephritis; PSGN, poststreptococcal glomerulonephritis; RBC, red blood cells; ROS, review of systems; SFLC, serum-free light chains; SPEP, serum protein electrophoresis; TMA, thrombotic microangiopathy; UA w/micro, Urinalysis with microscopy; UPEP, urine protein electrophoresis; US, ultrasound; WBC, white blood cells.

Table 3
Etiologies of glomerular diseases

Renal Disease	Causes
Minimal change disease	
Drugs	NSAIDs, interferon, gold, lithium
Allergy	Pollens, house dust, insect stings, immunizations
Malignancy	Hodgkin's diseases, mycosis fungoldes, chronic lymphocytic lymphoma
FSGS	
Primary (idiopathic)	
Secondary	
Genetic	Mutations in nephrin, mutations in podocin, mutations in α-actinin 4
Viral	HIV-1 (HIV-AN), parvovirus B19, SV40, CMV
Drug induced	Heroin, interferon, lithium, pamidronate, sirolimus
Adaptive, reduced renal mass	Oligomeganephronia, very low birth weight, unilateral renal agenesis, renal dysplasia, reflux nephropathy, sequelae to cortical necrosis, surgical renal ablation, chronic allograft nephropathy, advanced renal disease with reduced functioning nephrons
Adaptive, initially normal renal mass	Hypertension, atheroemboli or other acute vasoocclusive processes, obesity, increased less body mass, anabolic steroids, cyanotic congenital heart disease, Sickle cell anemia
MPGN	
Type 1 w/mixed cyroglobulinemia	Hepatitis C virus, bacterial endocarditis, chronic hepatitis B infection, SLE, Sjögren syndrome, CLL, non-Hodgkin's lymphoma
Type 1 w/o cryoglobulinemia	Endocarditis, abscess, infected ventriculoatrial shunt, hepatitis (B, C, G), HIV, Hantavirus, malaria, SLE-hypocomplementemic urticarial vasculitis, hereditary complement deficiencies (C1q, C2, C4, C3), acquired complement deficiency (presence of C4 nephritic factor), chronic liver disease, Sickle cell disease, CLL, lymphoma, thymoma, RCC
Dense deposit disease	A/w C3 neph, A/w factor H defect
MPGN type III	Secondary causes similar to MPGN type 1 (hepatitis C, B and other)
Membranous nephropathy	
Immune diseases	SLE, DM, RA, Hashimoto's disease, Grave's disease, MCTD, Sjögren syndrome, PBC, bullous pemphigoid, small bowel enteropathy syndrome, dermatitis herpetiformis, ankylosing spondylitis, graft-vs-host disease, GBS, bone marrow and stem cell transplant, anti-GBM and ANCA + crescentic GN
Infectious diseases	Hepatitis B, hepatitis C, syphilis, filariarsis, hydatid disease, schistosomiasis, malaria, leprosy
Drugs	Gold, penicillamine, NSAIDs, mercury, captopril, formaldehyde, hydrocarbons, bucillamine agents
Miscellaneous	Tumors, renal transplantation, sarcoidosis, Sickle cell disease, Kimura disease, angiofollicular lymph node hyperplasia

Abbreviations: CLL, chronic lymphocytic leukemia; CMV, cytomegalovirus; DM, diabetes mellitus; FSGS, focal segmental glomerulosclerosis; GBM, glomerular basement membrane; GBS, Guillain-Barre syndrome; GN, glomerulonephritis; HIV-AN, HIV-associated nephropathy; MCTD, mixed connective tissue disease; MPGN, membranoproliferative glomerulonephritis; NSAID, nonsteroidal anti-inflammatory drug; PBC, primary biliary cirrhosis; RA, rheumatoid arthritis; RCC, renal cell carcinoma; SLE, systemic lupus erythematosus.

Adapted from Floege J, Johnson RJ, Feehally J. Comprehensive clinical nephrology. 4th edition. St Louis (MO): Elsevier; 2010.

Case 1

A 69-year-old man with history of long-standing diabetes mellitus as well as diabetic microvascular complications (ie, diabetic retinopathy, diabetic neuropathy, and cardiac disease) is expected to have renal disease owing to diabetes as well. In this case, the patient may have nephrotic range proteinuria and some degree of renal insufficiency. The patient might not need a kidney biopsy if he or she meets the following conditions: He or she does not have history suggestive of other infectious or inflammatory processes, the review of systems is otherwise negative, urinary sediment is bland (no cells or casts), and the patient is up to date on routine cancer screenings.

DIABETIC NEPHROPATHY

Diabetes mellitus is the leading cause of ESRD in the United States. Diabetic nephropathy begins with microvascular damage followed by hyper-filtration early in the disease. Microalbuminuria is succeeded by macroalbuminuria and then slow progressive decline in GFR.[18] According to American Diabetes Association, urine albumin should be checked in type 1 diabetics 5 years after diagnosis and in type 2 diabetics at the time of diagnosis and should be monitored annually if negative and more often if abnormal. Hyperglycemia causes formation of glycation end products that deposit in the mesangium, where they cause direct mesangial expansion and irreversible injury over time. Hyperglycemia stimulates vascular endothelial growth factor, leading to endothelial injury and increases expression of transforming growth factor-β, which is profibrotic.[19,20] Thus, when renal ultrasonography shows normal sized or larger kidneys in the diabetic, it may be largely owing to mesangial expansion. The dilemma in diabetic nephropathy is that etiologies of other nephrotic range proteinuria may coexist. If clues that lead one to suspect nondiabetic nephropathy exist (acute onset of macroalbuminuria, urine sediment with RBCs that are isomorphic or dysmorphic, diabetes mellitus diagnosed <5 years without retinopathy or neuropathy, serologies positive for antinuclear antibody, hepatitis, or HIV), a biopsy is recommended.

Case 2

A 20-year-old Asian man with no significant previous medical history comes in with complaints of recent onset of diarrhea, joint pains, and skin lesions. Physical examination shows hypertension, palpable purpura, and abdominal tenderness. A basic metabolic panel shows normal electrolytes, blood urea nitrogen of 32, and creatinine of 1.8. A urinalysis showed ++ blood, ++++ protein, and 15 to 20 RBCs. Does this patient need a biopsy? If so, what would it likely reveal?

IMMUNOGLOBULIN A NEPHROPATHY

Immunoglobulin (Ig)A nephropathy occurs owing to the deposition of genetically induced galactose deficient IgA in the glomerular mesangium. The O-glycans of IgA1 hinge region in the heavy chain goes without galactosylation.[21] Relatives also with elevated galactose-deficient IgA1 levels can be without clinical or renal manifestations of the disease, which leads to the hypothesis that other factors contribute to the development of clinical disease.[21] Certain infections (viruses/bacteria) cause anti-glycan antibody formation that cross-reacts with galactose-deficient IgA, forming immune complexes, which then deposit and activate renal mesangial cells and complement system. This leads to mesangial hypercellularity, and apoptosis or expansion of mesangial matrix. Consequently, injury to both podocytes and proximal tubule epithelial cells occurs, with increased glomerular and interstitial scarring.[22]

The disease can recur after kidney transplantation, and resolution of IgA deposits have also been observed after transplantation of affected kidneys in ESRD patients with other primary renal pathologies.[23] Patients present with hematuria during recent or ongoing gastrointestinal infections or upper respiratory infections. This is different than post streptococcal infectious glomerulonephritis in which the time lag (1–6 weeks) from the original infection to renal disease suggests the time for the insulting immune process to occur. However, in IgA nephropathy, the symptoms are concurrent, as though owing to prior sensitization.

Patients with IgA nephropathy may present with hypertension, hematuria, or proteinuria alone, and the proteinuria might be either nephrotic or subnephrotic. Patients of a Pacific Asian origin have higher rates of progression to ESRD,[24] and there is lower incidence in African-American patients.[25] However, race cannot be reliably used to assist in diagnosis. Genetic testing has not been validated, and measuring serum IgA1 levels are not sensitive, because disease-free patients with galactose-deficient IgA may also have increased levels.[21] Ultimately, renal biopsy is needed to secure the diagnosis.

Worse outcomes are predicted clinically by sustained hypertension, declining renal function and proteinuria of more than 1 g,[26,27] and histologically via the Oxford classification method. This includes scoring for mesangial hypercellularity, glomerular sclerosis, endocapillary hypercellularity, and tubulointerstitial atrophy/fibrosis.[28] Immunofluorescence microscopy of kidney biopsy shows mainly galactose-deficient IgA deposits in the mesangium of the glomerulus, along with complement C3, properdin, IgG, and/or IgM. C4d, mannose-binding lectin, and terminal complement complex (C5b-C9).[29] Serum complement levels would be normal. There is usually mesangial cellular proliferation and thus mesangial matrix expansion. However, if blood pressure is controlled, proteinuria may be decreased to less than 1 g in 24 hours, and if there is no alteration in renal function, many nephrologists do not pursue a biopsy, preferring to monitor closely.

The patient in case 2 has Henoch–Schönlein purpura. Henoch–Schönlein purpura and IgA nephropathy represent a clinical spectrum of IgA pathology, and have the same renal biopsy findings.

Case 3

A 19-year-old African-American woman presents office with periorbital and facial swelling, as well as edema of the lower extremities. Physical examination shows hypertension and discoid lesions on the upper arms. Urine dipstick shows +++ RBCs and +++ protein. Urine microscopy shows dysmorphic RBCs and RBC casts. SSA turns the urine opaque white.

LUPUS NEPHRITIS

Systemic lupus erythematous may present with a variety of symptoms, including but not limited to malar rash, discoid lesions on the skin, oral ulcers, arthralgias, and serositis. Further blood work may show renal insufficiency, leukopenia, anemia, and thrombocytopenia. Proteinuria may range from nephritic to nephrotic range. Examination of urine sediment may show damaged or dysmorphic RBCs that have passed through the glomeruli. Antinuclear antibody and dsDNA antibody are usually positive, and the erythrocyte sedimentation rate is elevated. The histologic features on a renal biopsy confirm the diagnosis, as well as suggest the aggressiveness of the treatment.

FOCAL SEGMENTAL GLOMERULOSCLEROSIS

Focal segmental glomerulosclerosis (FSGS) is the most common primary glomerular disorder causing ESRD in the United States. This disease is defined by the histologic features on kidney biopsy, which shows focal (only certain glomeruli) segments (part of the glomerulus) with fibrosis and effacement of podocytes that lead to proteinuria. This disease can be categorized as primary/idiopathic or secondary, and then further categorized by varying pathologic features. Certain pathologic features are more suggestive of certain secondary causes (**Table 4**). FSGS is thought to occur owing to circulating permeability factors,[30] which seems to be removable by plasmapheresis.

Genetic abnormalities can lead to mutations of proteins that encode podocyte cell signaling and cell structure, leading to structural variability and an inability to endure external stimuli or sheer stress, which can over time cause podocyte malfunction.[12] Variations in the gene encoding apolipoprotein 1 have been associated with FSGS. This variant found in people of African descent provide resistance to Trypanosoma (sleeping sickness), which may explain why African Americans have been found to have an higher prevalence of FSGS than Caucasians.[31] Other genes implicated in primary FSGS are still being studied.

FSGS can occur owing to hyperfiltration in the glomerulus as compensation for decreased mass, which leads to intrarenal vasodilatation, increased capillary pressures, and increased plasma flow rates.[32] This in turn leads to hypertrophy of the glomeruli, causing the podocytes to stretch to cover the growing surface area. The renin–angiotensin–aldosterone system is also activated, which worsens proteinuria and sclerosis. In addition, angiotensin II itself can promote apoptosis in podocytes.[33]

Viruses like HIV can cause direct damage to both the glomerulus and tubular epithelial cells, causing the glomeruli to collapse. Thus, HIV-associated nephropathy is also known as collapsing FSGS. This form of FSGS is characteristic of HIV, but it is not unique only to viruses. It can also be caused by certain drugs. For example, pamidronate (an osteoclast inhibitor) can also cause proteinuria with a collapsing FSGS-like picture on kidney biopsy, which may or may not improve with withdrawal of the offending agent.[34]

CHRONIC KIDNEY DISEASE CLASSIFICATION AND PROTEINURIA

Categorizing the degree of proteinuria when classifying CKD was introduced with the release of KDIGO guidelines in 2012 (**Fig. 3**). Proteinuria is an earlier marker of CKD than the decline in eGFR, but there have been numerous studies that show a direct correlation between proteinuria and mortality owing to cardiovascular disease.[35] Within the CKD predialysis population, higher degrees of proteinuria alone within the same classification of eGFR have increased risk of death, myocardial infarction, and worsening of CKD.[36] In patients with type 2 diabetes, albuminuria has been associated with abnormal ventricular function.[37] These findings were consistent whether the cause of proteinuria was diabetic nephropathy or nondiabetic disease. Moreover, this relationship exists even when there is minimal albuminuria (<30 mg/dL).[18] When the findings of proteinuria are extrapolated to the general population with normal eGFR, increase in proteinuria (owing to any cause) leads to an increased risk in all-cause mortality, and especially in risk of cardiovascular death.[38]

This relationship of proteinuria and cardiovascular disease is thought to be multifactorial, involving insulin resistance, endothelial dysfunction, a prothrombotic state, and inflammation owing to the lack of nitric oxide being released by endothelial cells owing to inflammation.[39] These factors eventually lead to left ventricular dysfunction and coronary artery microthrombi. Recent review shows that adiponectin and activated

Table 4
Histologic subtypes of FSGS and its associations

Histologic Subtype of FSGS	Associations	Clinical Features
NOS	Primary or secondary (including genetic forms and other diverse secondary causes). Cross-sectional studies suggest this is the most common subtype. Other variants can evolve into FSGS (NOS) over time.	May present with nephrotic syndrome or subnephrotic proteinuria
Perihilar	Common in adaptive FSGS associated with obesity elevated lean body mass, reflux nephropathy, hypertensive nephrosclerosis, sickle cell anemia, and renal agenesis. Predisposition for vascular pole is probably owing to normally increased filtration pressures at the proximal apparent end of glomerular capillary bed, which are heightened under conditions of compensatory demand and vasodilatation of the afferent arteriole.	In adaptive FSGS, patients are more likely to present with subnephrotic proteinuria and normal serum albumin levels.
Cellular	Usually primary, but also seen in a variety of secondary forms. This is the least common variant. It is thought to represent an early stage in the evolution of sclerotic lesions.	Usually presents with nephrotic syndrome.
Tip	Usually primary. Probably mediated by physical stressors on the paratubular segment owing to the convergence of protein-rich filtrate on the tubular pole, causing shear stress and possible prolapse.	Usually presents with abrupt onset of nephrotic syndrome. More common in white race. Best prognosis, with highest rate of responsivity to glucocorticoids and lowest risk of progression.
Collapse	Primary or secondary to viruses: HIV-1, parvovirus B19, SV40, EBV, CMV, hemophagocytic syndrome. Drugs: pamidronate and interferon Vasoocclusive disease: Atheroemboli, calcineurin inhibitor nephrotoxicity, and chronic allograft nephropathy.	Most aggressive variant of primary FSGS with black racial predominance and severe nephrotic syndrome. Worst prognosis, with poor responsivity to glucocorticoids and rapid course to renal failure.

Abbreviations: CMV, cytomegalovirus; EBV, Epstein–Barr virus: FSGS, focal segmental glomerulosclerosis; NOS, not otherwise specified.
Adapted from D'Agati VD, Kaskel FJ, Falk RJ. Focal Segmental glomerulosclerosis. N Engl J Med 2011;365(25):2398–411; with permission.

protein kinase (AMPK) activation may provide renal protection against albuminuria via activation of anti-inflammatory, antifibrotic, and antioxidative pathways.[40] Adiponectin, released by adipose tissue, has been found to be elevated in the urine even before the presence of microalbuminuria, and suggests disease progression in CKD.[40,41] Reduced adiponectin levels are seen in insulin resistance, cardiovascular disease,

				Persistent albuminuria categories Description and range		
				A1	**A2**	**A3**
				Normal to mildly increased	Moderately increased	Severely increased
				<30 mg/g <3 mg/mmol	30-300 mg/g 3-30 mg/mmol	>300 mg/g >30 mg/mmol
GFR categories (mL/min/ 1.73 m²) Description and range	G1	Normal or high	≥90			
	G2	Mildly decreased	60-89			
	G3a	Mildly to moderately decreased	45-59			
	G3b	Moderately to severely decreased	30-44			
	G4	Severely decreased	15-29			
	G5	Kidney failure	<15			

Green: low risk (if no other markers of kidney disease, no CKD); Yellow: moderately increased risk; Orange: high risk; Red, very high risk.

Fig. 3. Prognosis of chronic kidney disease (CKD) by glomerular filtration rate (GFR) and albuminuria categories: Kidney Disease: Improving Global Outcomes (KDIGO) CKD Work Group, 2012. (*From* Kidney disease: Improving Global Outcomes (KDIGO) CKD Work Group. KDIGO 2012 clinical practice guideline for the evaluation and management of chronic kidney disease. Kidney Int 2013;3Suppl:1–150.)

and obesity-related kidney disease.[41] In knockout rat models, rats that lack the adiponectin gene expression were demonstrated to have proteinuria.[40] Moreover, rats that were induced to produce more adiponectin were found to have increased endothelial nitric oxide synthase messenger RNA levels.[42] Increase in nitric oxide production is also a regulatory mechanism of protein permeability in glomeruli.[43]

GENERAL ASPECTS OF THERAPY

The landscape of treatments for these glomerular lesions is changing steadily. Depending on the degree of proteinuria and histologic features, immunosuppressive or biologic agents (alkylating agents, purine synthesis inhibitors, calcineurin inhibitors, and CD-20 antibody) may be initiated, with or without steroids. However, there are some basic concepts of therapy that may be applied to most of them, if not all.

Diet

Patients should be prescribed a low-sodium diet. There are mixed opinions on dietary restriction of protein in the diet. On one hand, it is thought that increased protein intake might increase the workload of the glomerulus and thus accelerate disease progression. On the other hand, there is the concern that protein restriction might compromise nutritional status. However, there is plenty of evidence that, once renal replacement therapy is initiated, nutritional status (as measured by serum albumin) has an inverse correlation with morbidity and mortality; thus, greater protein consumption is recommended for dialysis patients.

Edema

The hallmark presentation of proteinuria is edema, especially in the nephrotic syndrome. Severe edema that compromises function should be treated aggressively with loop-blocking diuretics. This includes pulmonary edema, severe ascites, and peripheral edema. If the degree of compromise is life threatening, or response to loop blockade is blunted, then distal and/or proximal diuretics can be added in a process that has been called "sequential nephroplegia." By adding a thiazide-type diuretic to a loop blocker, any opportunity for the distal tubules to reabsorb salt and water is blunted, and true synergy can be achieved. In even more severe situations, the further addition of acetazolamide to block proximal tubular absorption can be attempted. However, when none of these measures is effective, the patient might need the intervention of ultrafiltration with or without dialysis.

On the other hand, lesser degrees of edema, for instance, moderate to mild peripheral edema only, can be treated less aggressively. The caveats are that aggressive diuresis with loop blockers may occur at the expense of intravascular volume, and result in pre-renal azotemia, or that electrolyte imbalances such as hypokalemia may supervene. These precautions have to guide diuretic therapy in any case. In all cases, salt restriction must be enforced.

Hypertension

Hypertension is a defining feature of the nephritic syndrome and a frequent concomitant of the nephrotic syndrome. The recent release of Eighth Joint National Committee (JNC 8) suggested that blood pressure reduction to a level less than 140/90 mm Hg might be adequate for most groups. Previously, National Kidney Foundation blood pressure recommendations for patients with renal disease was for a goal blood pressure of 130/80 or less, supported by the opinion that this lower goal will help to retard progression of kidney disease. Both of these recommendations are opinion based rather than truly evidence based. The ultimate goal is at the discretion of the clinician. Therapy should be initiated with an ACE inhibitor or angiotensin receptor blocker. These agents should even be considered in the absence of hypertension, owing to the beneficial effects on intrarenal hemodynamics. There is ample evidence that these drug classes should not be combined owing to hyperkalemia and increased incidence of acute kidney injury.[44,45] Usually, a diuretic is needed because proteinuric syndromes are associated with defects in sodium excretion. Unlike essential hypertension, the choice can be a loop blocker rather than a thiazide. The role of direct renin inhibition has not been well defined, although early evidence showed that this route could reduce proteinuria. However, given the current state of knowledge regarding combinations of renin–angiotensin–aldosterone system drugs, it is not recommended to use different classes of renin–angiotensin–aldosterone system blockade in conjunction with one another.[46]

Lipids

Most patients with proteinuria, whether nephrotic, subnephrotic, or nephritic, have some degree of lipid abnormality. Perhaps the highest levels of cholesterol in any nonfamilial dyslipidemia can be seen in the most florid cases of the nephrotic syndrome. Statin drugs are recommended for primary management of dyslipidemia, and for reduction of the cardiovascular risk that accompanies renal disease.[47] In addition, among the pleiotropic effects attributed to statins, evidence suggests that they may reduce proteinuria and mitigate glomerular damage.[19] Thus, high-potency statins such as atorvastatin or rosuvastatin should be recommended for patients with proteinuria.

Progression of Azotemia and Other Complications

In some patients, azotemia progresses relentlessly despite optimal treatment. For these patients, standard measures that would be taken for any other patient with progressive CKD should be put in place. These include attention to development of anemia, secondary hyperparathyroidism, and bone mineral disease, and as the eGFR falls below 20 mL/min, preparations for dialysis should begin. Patients with CKD usually have normal urine output when dialysis is initiated, but this falls off within weeks to months. It is only when oliguria supervenes that proteinuria diminishes.

Patients are also at increased risk for infections and thrombotic events owing to loss of immunologic proteins and anticoagulant factors. Low-dose aspirin is recommended to prevent thrombotic events in hypoalbuminemic patients.

SUMMARY

Although microalbuminuria without renal insufficiency is often ignored, it is an early and sensitive marker of renal dysfunction associated with long term complications. Early detection of nonbenign proteinuria and referral is thus important to prevent further disease progression and avoid possible complications associated with proteinuria.

ACKNOWLEDGMENTS

The data reported here have been supplied by the United States Renal Data System (USRDS). The interpretation and reporting of these data are the responsibility of the author(s) and in no way should be seen as an official policy or interpretation of the U.S. government. A. Incidence. Table A1.

REFERENCES

1. Clase CM, Gao P, Tobe SW, et al. Estimated glomerular filtration rate and albuminuria as predictors of outcomes in patients with high cardiovascular risk: a cohort study. Ann Intern Med 2011;154(5):310–8. Available at: http://www.ncbi.nlm.nih.gov/pubmed/21357908. Accessed November 24, 2013.
2. Bello AK, Hemmelgarn B, Lloyd A, et al. Associations among estimated glomerular filtration rate, proteinuria, and adverse cardiovascular outcomes. Clin J Am Soc Nephrol 2011;6(6):1418–26. Available at: http://www.pubmedcentral.nih.gov/articlerender.fcgi?artid=3109940&tool=pmcentrez&rendertype=abstract. Accessed November 24, 2013.
3. Astor BC, Matsushita K, Gansevoort RT, et al. Lower estimated glomerular filtration rate and higher albuminuria are associated with mortality and end-stage renal disease. A collaborative meta-analysis of kidney disease population cohorts. Kidney Int 2011;79(12):1331–40. Available at: http://www.ncbi.nlm.nih.gov/pubmed/21289598. Accessed November 24, 2013.
4. Kidney Disease: Improving Global Outcomes (KDIGO) CKD Work Group. KDIGO 2012 Clinical practice guideline for the evaluation and management of chronic kidney disease. Kidney Int 2013;3(Suppl):1–150.

5. US Renal Data System (USRDS). 2013 annual data report: atlas of chronic kidney disease and end-stage renal disease in the United States. Bethesda (MD): National Institutes of Health, National Institute of Diabetes and Digestive and Kidney Diseases; 2013.
6. Huisman RM. The deadly risk of late referral. Nephrol Dial Transplant 2004;19(9): 2175–80. Available at: http://www.ncbi.nlm.nih.gov/pubmed/15299096. Accessed December 14, 2013.
7. Tseng CL, Kern EF, Miller DR, et al. Survival benefit of nephrologic care in patients with diabetes mellitus and chronic kidney disease. Arch Intern Med 2008;168(1): 55–62. Available at: http://www.ncbi.nlm.nih.gov/pubmed/18195196.
8. Rettig RA, Norris K, Nissenson AR. Chronic kidney disease in the United States: a public policy imperative. Clin J Am Soc Nephrol 2008;3(6):1902–10. Available at: http://www.ncbi.nlm.nih.gov/pubmed/18922986. Accessed December 14, 2013.
9. Byron A, Randles MJ, Humphries JD, et al. Glomerular cell cross-talk influences composition and assembly of extracellular matrix. J Am Soc Nephrol 2014;25(5): 953–66. Available at: http://www.ncbi.nlm.nih.gov/pubmed/24436469. Accessed February 5, 2014.
10. Floege J, Johnson RJ, Feehally J, editors. Comprehensive clinical nephrology. 4th edition. St Louis (MO): Elsevier; 2010.
11. Rose BD, Post TW. Clinical physiology of acid-base and electrolyte disorders. In: Wonsciewics M, McCullough K, Davis K, editors. Clinical physiology of acid-base and electrolyte disorders. 5th edition. McGraw Hill; 2001. p. 24–8, 99.
12. D'Agati VD, Kaskel FJ, Falk RJ. Focal Segmental Glomerulosclerosis. N Engl J Med 2011;365(25):2398–411. http://dx.doi.org/10.1056/NEJMra1106556.
13. Rampoldi L, Scolari F, Amoroso A, et al. The rediscovery of uromodulin (Tamm-Horsfall protein): from tubulointerstitial nephropathy to chronic kidney disease. Kidney Int 2011;80(4):338–47. Available at: http://www.ncbi.nlm.nih.gov/pubmed/21654721. Accessed February 5, 2014.
14. Chotayaporn T, Kasitanon N, Sukitawut W, et al. Comparison of proteinuria determination by urine dipstick, spot urine protein creatinine index, and urine protein 24 hours in lupus patients. J Clin Rheumatol 2011;17(3). Available at: http://journals.lww.com/jclinrheum/Fulltext/2011/04000/Comparison_of_Proteinuria_Determination_by_Urine.3.aspx. Accessed November 20, 2013.
15. Wills MR, McGowan GK. The reliability of the Albustix test for proteinuria. J Clin Pathol 1963;16(5):487. Available at: http://jcp.bmj.com/cgi/doi/10.1136/jcp.16.5.487. Accessed November 19, 2013.
16. Pugia MJ, Lott JA, Profitt JA, et al. High-sensitivity dye binding assay for albumin in urine. J Clin Lab Anal 1999;13(4):180–7. Available at: http://www.ncbi.nlm.nih.gov/pubmed/10414598. Accessed February 5, 2014.
17. Sethi S, Fervenza FC. Membranoproliferative glomerulonephritis–a new look at an old entity. N Engl J Med 2012;366(12):1119–31. Available at: http://www.ncbi.nlm.nih.gov/pubmed/22435371.
18. Gerstein HC, Mann JF, Yi Q, et al. Albuminuria and risk of cardiovascular events, death, and heart failure in diabetic and nondiabetic individuals. JAMA 2001; 286(4):421–6. Available at: http://www.ncbi.nlm.nih.gov/pubmed/11466120. Accessed January 28, 2014.
19. Dworacka M, Krzyżagórska E, Wesołowska A, et al. Statins in low doses reduce VEGF and bFGF serum levels in patients with type 2 diabetes mellitus. Pharmacology 2014;93(1–2):32–8. Available at: http://www.ncbi.nlm.nih.gov/pubmed/24434301. Accessed February 8, 2014.

20. Lee HS. Pathogenic role of TGF-β in the progression of podocyte diseases. Histol Histopathol 2011;26(1):107–16. Available at: http://www.ncbi.nlm.nih.gov/pubmed/21117032. Accessed February 8, 2014.
21. Gharavi AG, Moldoveanu Z, Wyatt RJ, et al. Aberrant IgA1 glycosylation is inherited in familial and sporadic IgA nephropathy. J Am Soc Nephrol 2008;19(5):1008–14. Available at: http://www.pubmedcentral.nih.gov/articlerender.fcgi?artid=2386728&tool=pmcentrez&rendertype=abstract. Accessed January 17, 2014.
22. Lai KN. Pathogenesis of IgA nephropathy. Nat Rev Nephrol 2012;8(5):275–83. Available at: http://www.ncbi.nlm.nih.gov/pubmed/22430056. Accessed January 17, 2014.
23. Ji S, Liu M, Chen J, et al. The fate of glomerular mesangial IgA deposition in the donated kidney after allograft transplantation. Clin Transplant 2004;18(5):536–40. Available at: http://www.ncbi.nlm.nih.gov/pubmed/15344956. Accessed January 19, 2014.
24. Barbour SJ, Cattran DC, Kim SJ, et al. Individuals of Pacific Asian origin with IgA nephropathy have an increased risk of progression to end-stage renal disease. Kidney Int 2013;84(5):1017–24. Available at: http://www.ncbi.nlm.nih.gov/pubmed/23739233. Accessed January 16, 2014.
25. Kiryluk K, Li Y, Sanna-Cherchi S, et al. Geographic differences in genetic susceptibility to IgA nephropathy: GWAS replication study and geospatial risk analysis. PLoS Genet 2012;8(6):e1002765. Available at: http://www.pubmedcentral.nih.gov/articlerender.fcgi?artid=3380840&tool=pmcentrez&rendertype=abstract. Accessed January 19, 2014.
26. Shen P, He L, Huang D. Clinical course and prognostic factors of clinical early IgA nephropathy. Neth J Med 2008;66(6):242–7. Available at: http://www.ncbi.nlm.nih.gov/pubmed/18689907. Accessed January 18, 2014.
27. Berthoux F, Mohey H, Laurent B, et al. Predicting the risk for dialysis or death in IgA nephropathy. J Am Soc Nephrol 2011;22(4):752–61. Available at: http://www.pubmedcentral.nih.gov/articlerender.fcgi?artid=3065230&tool=pmcentrez&rendertype=abstract. Accessed January 19, 2014.
28. Roberts IS. Oxford classification of immunoglobulin A nephropathy: an update. Curr Opin Nephrol Hypertens 2013;22(3):281–6. Available at: http://www.ncbi.nlm.nih.gov/pubmed/23518465. Accessed January 17, 2014.
29. Wyatt RJ, Julian B. IgA nephropathy. N Engl J Med 2013;368(25):2402–14. Available at: http://www.ncbi.nlm.nih.gov/pubmed/23782179. Accessed November 10, 2013.
30. McCarthy ET, Sharma M, Savin VJ. Circulating permeability factors in idiopathic nephrotic syndrome and focal segmental glomerulosclerosis. Clin J Am Soc Nephrol 2010;5(11):2115–21. Available at: http://www.ncbi.nlm.nih.gov/pubmed/20966123. Accessed January 14, 2014.
31. Genovese G, Friedman DJ, Ross MD, et al. Association of trypanolytic ApoL1 variants with kidney disease in African Americans. Science 2010;329(5993):841–5. Available at: http://www.pubmedcentral.nih.gov/articlerender.fcgi?artid=2980843&tool=pmcentrez&rendertype=abstract. Accessed January 5, 2014.
32. Rennke HG, Klein PS. Pathogenesis and significance of nonprimary focal and segmental glomerulosclerosis. Am J Kidney Dis 1989;13(6):443–56. Available at: http://www.ncbi.nlm.nih.gov/pubmed/2658558. Accessed January 6, 2014.
33. Shankland SJ. The podocyte's response to injury: role in proteinuria and glomerulosclerosis. Kidney Int 2006;69(12):2131–47. Available at: http://www.ncbi.nlm.nih.gov/pubmed/16688120. Accessed January 6, 2014.

34. ten Dam MA, Hilbrands LB, Wetzels JF. Nephrotic syndrome induced by pamidronate. Med Oncol 2011;28(4):1196–200. Available at: http://www.ncbi.nlm.nih.gov/pubmed/20865462. Accessed January 15, 2014.

35. Currie G, Delles C. Proteinuria and its relation to cardiovascular disease. Int J Nephrol Renovasc Dis 2013;7:13–24. Available at: http://www.pubmedcentral.nih.gov/articlerender.fcgi?artid=3873205&tool=pmcentrez&rendertype=abstract. Accessed January 27, 2014.

36. Hemmelgarn BR, Manns BJ, Lloyd A, et al. Relation between kidney function, proteinuria, and adverse outcomes. JAMA 2010;303(5):423–9. Available at: http://www.ncbi.nlm.nih.gov/pubmed/20124537. Accessed January 28, 2014.

37. Liu JE, Robbins DC, Palmieri V, et al. Association of albuminuria with systolic and diastolic left ventricular dysfunction in type 2 diabetes: the Strong Heart Study. J Am Coll Cardiol 2003;41(11):2022–8. Available at: http://www.ncbi.nlm.nih.gov/pubmed/12798576. Accessed January 29, 2014.

38. Hillege HL, Fidler V, Diercks GF, et al. Urinary albumin excretion predicts cardiovascular and noncardiovascular mortality in general population. Circulation 2002; 106(14):1777–82. Available at: http://www.ncbi.nlm.nih.gov/pubmed/12356629. Accessed January 28, 2014.

39. Stehouwer CD, Henry RM, Dekker JM, et al. Microalbuminuria is associated with impaired brachial artery, flow-mediated vasodilation in elderly individuals without and with diabetes: further evidence for a link between microalbuminuria and endothelial dysfunction–the Hoorn Study. Kidney Int 2004;92(Suppl):S42–4. Available at: http://www.ncbi.nlm.nih.gov/pubmed/15485416. Accessed January 30, 2014.

40. Christou GA, Kiortsis D. The role of adiponectin in renal physiology and development of albuminuria. J Endocrinol 2014;221(2):R49–61. Available at: http://www.ncbi.nlm.nih.gov/pubmed/24464020. Accessed January 29, 2014.

41. Sweiss N, Sharma K. Adiponectin effects on the kidney. Best Pract Res Clin Endocrinol Metab 2014;28(1):71–9. Available at: http://www.ncbi.nlm.nih.gov/pubmed/24417947. Accessed January 31, 2014.

42. Nakamaki S, Satoh H, Kudoh A, et al. Adiponectin reduces proteinuria in streptozotocin-induced diabetic Wistar rats. Exp Biol Med (Maywood) 2011; 236(5):614–20. Available at: http://www.ncbi.nlm.nih.gov/pubmed/21521713. Accessed January 30, 2014.

43. Datta PK, Sharma M, Duann P, et al. Effect of nitric oxide synthase inhibition on proteinuria in glomerular immune injury. Exp Biol Med (Maywood) 2006;231(5): 576–84. Available at: http://www.ncbi.nlm.nih.gov/pubmed/16636306. Accessed January 30, 2014.

44. Fried LF, Emanuele N, Zhang JH, et al. Combined angiotensin inhibition for the treatment of diabetic nephropathy. N Engl J Med 2013;369(20):1892–903. Available at: http://www.ncbi.nlm.nih.gov/pubmed/24206457. Accessed February 3, 2014.

45. Mann JF, Schmieder RE, McQueen M, et al. Renal outcomes with telmisartan, ramipril, or both, in people at high vascular risk (the ONTARGET study): a multicentre, randomised, double-blind, controlled trial. Lancet 2008;372(9638): 547–53. Available at: http://www.ncbi.nlm.nih.gov/pubmed/18707986. Accessed February 9, 2014.

46. Parving HH, Brenner BM, McMurray JJ, et al. Cardiorenal end points in a trial of aliskiren for type 2 diabetes. N Engl J Med 2012;367(23):2204–13. Available at: http://www.ncbi.nlm.nih.gov/pubmed/23121378. Accessed February 3, 2014.

47. Valdivielso P, Moliz M, Valera A, et al. Atorvastatin in dyslipidaemia of the nephrotic syndrome. Nephrology (Carlton) 2003;8(2):61–4. Available at: http://www.ncbi.nlm.nih.gov/pubmed/15012735. Accessed February 9, 2014.

Work-up of Hematuria

Saifullah N. Kazi, MBBS, MD[a,*], Robert L. Benz, MD[b]

KEYWORDS

- Hematuria • Urinary abnormalities • Urinalysis • Renal stones
- Malignancy of urinary tract • Glomerulonephritis

KEY POINTS

- Hematuria is a common clinical manifestation of diseases affecting the urinary system. However, it may not represent any underlying disease and may be of no clinical significance, especially when it is transient in young adult patients. On the other hand, it may represent underlying malignancy in older patients, even if transient.
- Detection of hematuria in the appropriate clinical setting and further investigation based on the individual clinical scenario helps establishing the correct diagnosis and guide further management.
- Discolored urine may appear as gross hematuria, but may actually reflect other etiologies including beeturia, myoglobinuria or hemoglobinuria. The key to diagnosis involves use of dipstick in the spun ruine examining the supernatant versus the sediment appearance.

INTRODUCTION

Presence of blood in the urine is known as hematuria. It can be divided into macroscopic hematuria, which is grossly visible, or microscopic hematuria, which is detectable only on urine chemical (dipstick) or microscopic examination of centrifuged urinary sediment. Hematuria can be defined by the presence of greater than two red blood cells (RBCs) per high power field (HPF) on microscopic examination of urinary sediment.[1–4]

According to the US Preventive Services Task Force on Periodic Health Examination, routine screening for hematuria is not indicated because it is not cost effective and the diseases causing it do not meet the criteria for screening. The prevalence of undetected, asymptomatic, and early disease is relatively low. There is little evidence that hematuria is a sensitive indicator for localized disease or that early treatment of a local disease results in a better prognosis. In one study, results of a urinary dipstick test in more than 10,000 adult men undergoing health screening were found to have positive test in about 2.5% of the cases. Twenty-five percent of those who underwent further investigation had cystoscopic abnormalities, including bladder neoplasms in two of them.[5]

Disclosures: None.
[a] Lankenau Medical Center and Research Institute, 100 E Lancaster Avenue, Wynnewood, PA 19096, USA; [b] Division of Nephrology, Main Line Health System, Lankenau Medical Center, Thomas Jefferson University Medical Center, Lankenau Institute of Medical Research, 100 East Lancaster Avenue, Wynnewood, PA 19096, USA
* Corresponding author.
E-mail address: docsaifnk@yahoo.co.in

Prim Care Clin Office Pract 41 (2014) 737–748
http://dx.doi.org/10.1016/j.pop.2014.08.007   primarycare.theclinics.com

BACKGROUND INCIDENCE

About 10% of men older than age 50 tested weekly for 3 months had evidence of hematuria.

CLASSIFICATION

Hematuria can be classified into several different categories. Based on site of origin it can be classified as glomerular versus nonglomerular. Based on location it can be classified as upper urinary tract (collecting ducts, calices, renal pelvis, and ureters) versus lower urinary tract (bladder and urethra). It can be intermittent versus persistent hematuria. It can be true hematuria versus discolored urine.

DIAGNOSIS

Hematuria can be detected by the urine dipstick test. Gross hematuria with blood clots almost never indicates glomerular bleeding; rather, it suggests a postrenal source in the urinary collecting system.[6] A single urinalysis showing microscopic hematuria is not uncommon and can be seen with menstruation and sometimes as cyclic hematuria caused by endometriosis, viral illness, allergy, exercise, or mild trauma. Persistent or significant hematuria as defined by more than three RBCs per HPF on three urinalyses or a single urinalysis with more than 100 RBCs per HPF or gross hematuria identified significant renal or urologic lesions (found in 9.1% of more than 1000 patients tested).[6]

The suspicion for urogenital neoplasms in patients with isolated hematuria increases with advancing age. Neoplasms are rare in the pediatric population, and isolated hematuria is more likely to be associated with a congenital anomaly or idiopathic. Acute cystitis and urethritis in women can cause gross hematuria.[6]

Urine dipstick is at least as sensitive as urinary sediment inspection by microscopy. It has more false-positives but it is unusual for false-negatives to occur. Urine dipstick detects hemoglobin, which is positive even if RBC lysis occurs because of dilute urine or prolonged standing of the specimen. Negative dipstick reliably excludes hematuria. Microscopic hematuria may be no more common in men with than without benign prostatic hyperplasia. The diagnosis of benign prostatic hyperplasia alone should not preclude thorough evaluation of underlying cause.

Urine Microscopy

Urine sediment inspection by light microscopy is very helpful in establishing the cause of hematuria. When urine is observed through phase-contrast microscopy various elements are observed. These are quantified as number per microscopic field. Based on urinary findings that accompany the observation of hematuria, and in the appropriate clinical setting, one can make a correct diagnosis.

Cells

Erythrocytes

There are two main forms of urinary erythrocytes: isomorphic, with regular shapes and contour derived from urinary excretory system; and dysmorphic, with irregular shapes and contours of glomerular origin. RBCs that reach the urine from the glomerulus become dysmorphic as they experience rapid and dramatic osmolar changes affecting the cell membrane on the course through the nephron. The term isolated hematuria refers to having only RBCs (no other blood cell types) in the urine.

Leukocytes
Neutrophils are the most frequently found leukocytes in urine. They represent lower or upper urinary tract inflammation or infection, but may also be the result of genital secretions especially in young women.

Renal tubular epithelial cells
These cells are derived from the exfoliation of tubular epithelium. They are a marker of tubular damage and found in acute kidney injury, acute interstitial nephritis, and acute cellular rejection of a renal allograft.

Squamous cells
These cells are derived from the urethra or from external genitalia. They indicate contamination from genital secretion.

Casts

Casts are molds of the lumen of tubules, composed of the precipitation of a protein secreted by tubular epithelial cells called uromodulin, previously known as Tamm-Horsfall protein. This precipitation occurs especially when urine is concentrated or alkaline. Casts are described by particles or cells flowing through the tubules that might become trapped in the precipitate. This observation enables one to characterize their role in diagnosis of renal disease.

Hyaline casts
These are colorless with a low refractive index, and contain no formed elements or cellular debris. They are simply the precipitation of uromodulin in the form of the tubular lumen. Hyaline casts may occur in normal urine, especially in volume depletion in which urine is concentrated and acidic, both favoring precipitation of uromodulin protein (eg, in prerenal azotemia).

Granular casts
Granular casts can be either finely or coarsely granular. They are typical of renal failure but not more specific. They result from necrotic renal tubular epithelial cells that fall into the tubular lumen and take on the shape of tubular lumen.

Waxy casts
These casts derive their name from their appearances, which is similar to melted wax. They are typical of patients with renal failure.

Erythrocyte casts
Erythrocyte casts may contain a few erythrocytes or so many that the matrix cannot be identified. The finding of these casts indicates hematuria of glomerular origin.

White blood cell casts
These contain variable numbers of polymorphonuclear leukocytes. They are found in acute pyelonephritis and acute interstitial nephritis, and may appear in chronic disease.

Crystals

Uric acid crystals
Uric acid crystals have an amber color and a wide spectrum of appearances including rhomboid and barrels. They are found only in acidic urine (pH ≤ 5.8).

Calcium oxalate crystal
There are two types of calcium oxalate crystals. Bihydrated crystals most often have a bipyramidal appearance. Monohydrated crystals are ovoid, dumbbell-shaped, or biconcave disks.

Cystine crystals

These crystals occur in patients with cystinuria and are hexagonal plates with irregular sides that are often heaped one on the other. This is an uncommon congenital finding.

CAUSES

Hematuria can be a symptom of an underlying disease, some of which are life threatening. Based on clinical presentation the causes of hematuria can be divided as most common, less common, and rare.

The most common causes include the following:

- Urinary tract infections
- Bladder stone, ureteral stone, and kidney stones
- Benign prostatic hyperplasia

The less common causes of hematuria include the following:

- Renal parenchymal diseases, such as glomerulonephritis and interstitial nephritis
- Trauma
- Cancers of urinary bladder and renal cell carcinoma
- Inflammation of the prostate, such as prostatitis

Rare causes of hematuria include the following:

- Loin pain–hematuria syndrome
- Exercise-induced hematuria
- Transient microscopic hematuria of elderly
- Arteriovenous malformations
- Nutcracker syndrome
- Analgesic nephropathy
- Alport syndrome
- Thin basement membrane disease

In the next sections individual disease associated with hematuria and their other manifestations that aid in establishing the diagnosis are discussed.

Renal Stones

Renal and ureteral stones are a common problem found in primary care practice. Patients may be asymptomatic or symptomatic with renal colic and hematuria. A total of 80% of patients with renal calculi have calcium-based stones, most of which are composed of calcium oxalate. Gross or microscopic hematuria occurs in most patients with symptomatic renal calculi. Hematuria is the single most discriminating predictor of a kidney stone in patients with unilateral flank pain. Noncontrast stone protocol computed tomography (CT) scan of the abdomen is diagnostic of renal or ureteral calculi. This protocol, also called a helical CT, avoids the use of contrast and provides high definition with fine cuts of 3- to 5-mm thickness.

In a primary care practice it is important to recognize the subset of patients with hematuria who fall into the category of having glomerulonephritis and referring them to a nephrologist for collaborative management. Gross hematuria with blood clots almost never indicates glomerular bleeding; rather, it suggests a postrenal source in the urinary collecting system. This is because kidneys contain enzymes that breakdown the clots, thus preventing clots from forming in the nephron.

Alport Syndrome (Hereditary Nephritis)

This is an X-linked dominant hereditary disease characterized by isolated persistent hematuria, deafness, and family history of chronic renal failure, which occurs primarily in males. It is caused by an abnormality in alpha 5 chain of type IV collagen.

Thin Basement Membrane Disease

This disease also manifests with persistent and isolated hematuria. It is an autosomal-dominant disease with strong family history. It typically has a benign course but can occasionally progress to chronic kidney disease.[3]

IgA Nephropathy

This condition presents with recurrent episodes of gross hematuria typically 1 to 3 days following upper respiratory tract infection. Urine color may return to normal within few days but microscopic hematuria may persist indefinitely with exacerbations of gross hematuria episodically.

Exercise-Induced Hematuria

This can be caused by direct trauma as may happen in long-distance runners causing trauma to urinary bladder because of repeated up and down motions. It can also be seen in such sports as rowing and swimming.[7–9]

About 30% of long-distance runners have gross hematuria with dysmorphic RBCs by microscopy along with RBC casts and mild proteinuria.[10] It is a benign condition with no long-term morbidity. Hematuria typically resolves within days of discontinuation of running.

Hematuria Following Upper Respiratory Tract Infection

Hematuria following upper respiratory tract infection is caused by immune complex deposition within glomeruli. Prospective studies reveal asymptomatic hematuria in 3.8% of patients after nonstreptococcal upper respiratory tract infection[11] and 8% following Group A β-hemolytic streptococci.[12] The causes for hematuria after an upper respiratory tract infection include poststreptococcal glomerulonephritis, IgA nephropathy, nonspecific mesangioproliferative glomerulonephritis, and acute allergic interstitial nephritis.

Poststreptococcal Glomerulonephritis

This is induced by infection with specific nephritogenic strains of Group A β-hemolytic streptococci, such as type 12 and type 49. Children younger than 7 years old are at greatest risk. The latent period typically is 10 days with pharyngitis to 21 days with impetigo. Patients can present with asymptomatic hematuria to full nephritic syndrome with red-brown urine, proteinuria (possibly nephrotic range), edema, hypertension, and even acute renal failure. It can be diagnosed by throat culture. By streptococcus diagnosis panel, only 50% have elevated ASO positive with impetigo. Low complements are seen. Poststreptococcal glomerulonephritis resolves gradually with renal function improving in 1 to 2 weeks. Complement levels return to normal within 6 weeks, and hematuria clears within 6 months. Remission is normal, and recurrence of the disease is rare.

Nonspecific Mesangioproliferative Glomerulonephritis

This occurs in up to 4% of patients with nonstreptococcal upper respiratory disease. Typically microscopic hematuria with RBC casts is seen. Hematuria resolves within several months. It has an excellent prognosis.

NONGLOMERULAR CAUSES

Discussed next are conditions affecting kidneys that are nonglomerular in origin but that still present with hematuria.

Sickle Cell Disease and Trait

Sickle cell disease is an autosomal-recessive inherited disorder, predominantly of African or African-American origin. Hematuria is a common clinical manifestation in sickle cell anemia and occurs in 3% to 4% of subjects with sickle cell trait at some point. There is often persistent microscopic hematuria with episodic gross hematuria. Urinary erythrocytes are isomorphic, but sickled erythrocytes are occasionally found in the urine.

Acute Allergic Interstitial Nephritis

Acute interstitial nephritis is a renal disease that is characterized by inflammatory infiltrates in the renal interstitium. It is not necessarily caused by upper respiratory tract infection but could occur because of antibiotic therapy for the underlying infection. Its onset is usually 5 to 10 days postantibiotic exposure but may occur sooner in patients previously exposed to the same antibiotics. Many other drugs besides antibiotics may also be implicated. Patients may present with acute kidney injury, sterile pyuria, and eosinophilia with eosinophiluria.

Transient Hematuria of the Elderly

This has more serious implications because of the risk of underlying serious disease with 2.4% incidence of malignancy (kidney, bladder, prostate). Ultrasound is best for screening renal tumors, whereas cystoscopy is best for bladder and prostate cancer.

Medullary Sponge Kidney

Medullary sponge kidney is a disorder characterized by dilated medullary and papillary collecting ducts that give the renal medulla a "spongy" appearance. It is asymptomatic unless complicated by nephrolithiasis, hematuria, or infection. Hematuria is intermittent and recurrent.

Tumors

Suspicion for malignancy in patients presenting with hematuria is of great concern. Recognizing appropriate sets of patients belonging to a high-risk group and ordering appropriate imaging studies facilitates management and expedites diagnosis.

Malignancy as a cause of hematuria is more common in males. More than 8% of healthy males age greater than 50 years with asymptomatic, isolated hematuria detected by dipstick had urinary tract malignancy.[13] Some of the cancers known to cause hematuria include renal cell carcinoma and cancers of urinary bladder and prostate.

Renal cell carcinoma

This can present with a range of symptoms. However, most patients are asymptomatic until the disease is advanced. Hematuria is included in the classic triad of renal cell carcinoma along with flank pain and palpable abdominal mass,[14] but this triad is present in less than 10% of diagnosed patients.

Bladder cancers

This typically presents with painless hematuria, although irritative voiding symptoms, such as urinary frequency, urgency, and dysuria, can be initial manifestations.

Hematuria in bladder cancer is the most common presenting symptom and is usually intermittent, gross, painless, and present through the course of micturition.

Prostate cancer

Hematuria is an uncommon presentation of prostate cancer. However, the presence of hematuria in elderly men should prompt consideration of prostate cancer in the differential diagnosis. Irritative voiding symptoms, such as urinary frequency, urgency, nocturia, and hesitancy, are more common.

RARE MISCELLANEOUS ETIOLOGIES

Some of the rare causes of hematuria are hereditary hemorrhagic telangectasias, radiation cystitis, schistosomiasis, arteriovenous malformations, nutcracker syndrome, and the loin pain–hematuria syndrome.

Arteriovenous Malformation

This can be congenital or acquired hematuria. The primary presenting sign is gross hematuria, but high-output heart failure and hypertension also may be seen.[14] Irregular filling defects by intravenous pyelogram caused by compression of the renal pelvis or the calyx are seen. This can be confirmed with arteriogram or computerized axial tomography scan. There are several therapeutic options. Treatment options include embolization or ablation or surgery.[15]

Loin Pain–Hematuria

This is a poorly defined disorder. Flank pain is usually severe and unrelenting. Microscopic examination of the urine reveals dysmorphic RBCs suggesting glomerular origin.[16,17] There is high incidence of other psychosomatic symptoms.[18] There is some possibility of underlying thin basement membrane disease.[19] Treatment strategies include possible benefit with angiotensin-converting enzyme inhibitors, which act by reducing intraglomerular pressure. Pain control with analgesics, nerve blocks, and transplantation has been successful.

Nutcracker Syndrome

The nutcracker syndrome refers to compression of the left renal vein between the aorta and proximal superior mesenteric vein. It can cause either gross or microscopic hematuria. It is usually asymptomatic but can sometimes be associated with loin pain. The diagnosis is usually made by using Doppler ultrasonography of left renal vein diameter and peak velocity or by magnetic resonance angiography or renal venography.[20–22]

INITIAL EVALUATION OF HEMATURIA

Look for any clues from the history and physical examination. Try to distinguish between glomerular and extraglomerular causes of hematuria. This can be done by subjecting urine to centrifugation and taking the sediment and observing it under light microscope for the presence of dysmorphic RBC (hallmark of glomerulonephritis).

Changes in the shapes of the RBCs can be caused by changes in pH and osmolarity as RBC travels through distal tubules of nephrons. However, there is significant observer variability in detecting dysmorphic RBCs, especially if phase-contrast microscopy is not available.[23]

Phase-contrast microscopy is an optical microscopy technique that converts phase shifts in the light passing through a transparent specimen to brightness changes in the image. Phase shifts themselves are invisible, but become more visible when shown as brightness variation.

Another important step is to differentiate between persistent hematuria and intermittent hematuria. Certain clues for the diagnosis include the following:

- Concurrent pyuria or dysuria could suggest urinary tract infection
- Recent upper respiratory tract infection could suggest the possibilities of post-streptococcal glomerulonephritis or IgA nephropathy
- Strong family history may be suggestive of hereditary nephritis or polycystic kidney disease
- Unilateral flank pain is suggestive of ureteral obstruction with a stone or blood clot or loin pain–hematuria syndrome
- Symptoms of benign prostatic hyperplasia in men
- Recent vigorous exercise
- History of bleeding disorders or use of anticoagulants
- Menstrual cycles in females causing cyclic hematuria
- Family history of sickle cell disease

Microscopic hematuria that occurs in patients who are taking anticoagulants requires urologic and nephrologic evaluations regardless of the type or level of anticoagulation therapy.

Three Tube Test

This test involves collection and comparison of three specimens: (1) initial urine sample, (2) midstream urine sample, and (3) terminal urine sample. Initial urine sample with hematuria suggests urethral cause; terminal hematuria is more suggestive of bladder trigone lesion; and uniform hematuria is suggestive of renal, ureteric, or diffuse bladder pathologies.

Renal Biopsy

Renal biopsy is rarely indicated for isolated glomerular hematuria. In a study of 111 patients with isolated hematuria, 75 had biopsy.[24] After 3.5 years of follow-up of 85 patients, three developed proteinuria (IgA glomerulonephritis) and one developed proteinuria with chronic renal insufficiency (membranoproliferative). Management of these patients is not usually affected by the results of biopsy. If renal biopsy is attempted on these patients, the typical findings are normal renal parenchyma, IgA nephropathy, thin basement disease (benign familial hematuria), mild nonspecific glomerular abnormalities, and hereditary nephritis.[18]

Renal biopsy also has no role in patients with nonglomerular hematuria. These patients need thorough evaluation with imaging and/or cystoscopy particularly to rule out malignancy.

An important indication for performing a renal biopsy in patients with isolated glomerular hematuria is to determine the presence of factors for progressive disease, such as tubulointerstitial atrophy or fibrosis. This information along with the presence of proteinuria and/or rising serum creatinine helps determine prognosis.[24–26]

Consider renal biopsy if there is progressive worsening of renal function, increasing protein excretion, or presence of cellular casts.

Urine Cytology

The sensitivity of urine cytology is greatest for carcinoma of the bladder with approximate sensitivity of 90%. By comparison, sensitivity for upper tract transitional cell carcinoma is limited, with the reported false-negative rate being 65% (and as high as 96% with low-grade tumors).[23,27] It is usually obtained before cystoscopy, which should be performed in patients at risk for malignancy.

Role of Radiologic Testing

There is no single gold standard test for imaging in hematuria. Most physicians begin with ultrasound evaluation of the kidneys, ureters, and bladder. Multidetector CT urography is the preferred imaging study in patients with otherwise unexplained hematuria.[27] Other imaging modalities include intravenous pyelogram, retrograde pyelogram, ultrasonography, magnetic resonance imaging, magnetic resonance urography, and conventional CT scanning.

Ultrasound and intravenous urogram generate criteria identifying morphologic changes in the kidneys and collecting system. Although the presence of masses is established with reasonable accuracy, these methods do not provide criteria for tissue characterization. Therefore, the use of these modalities does not exclude the need for additional imaging studies. In addition, the sensitivities and specificities of ultrasonography and intravenous urogram are such that the possibility of missed diagnoses is significant.[22] Both of these issues are avoided with the use of CT urography and magnetic resonance imaging urography, two modalities that have been developed and refined during the last decade. CT urography provides a detailed anatomic depiction of the urinary tract but has higher radiation exposure. The average contrast dose in contrast-enhanced CT urography is more than double that of intravenous pyelogram.[28] Magnetic resonance urography, although possibly providing less anatomic detail, has the advantage of avoiding the use of ionizing radiation.[29]

Intravenous pyelogram may be reasonable to diagnose medullary sponge kidney in a young adult. Ultrasound is commonly used to rule out mass lesions, stones, or polycystic kidney disease. Computerized axial tomography scans are usually not indicated as initial work-up.

Cystoscopy

This is usually done in patients with unexplained hematuria with negative ultrasound or intravenous pyelogram. Yield is low in men age younger than 40 years and low-risk women. Men older than 50 years of age are considered high risk for malignancy, as are those with a history of smoking, exposure to dyes, phenactin, cyclophosphamide, and analgesic abuse.

Cystoscopy should be performed on all patients who present with risk factors for urinary tract malignancies.[30] Common risk factors for urinary tract malignancy in asymptomatic microscopic hematuria include the following:

- Male gender
- Age (>35 years)
- Past or current smoking
- Occupational or other exposure to chemicals or dyes (benzenes or aromatic amines)
- Analgesic abuse
- History of gross hematuria
- History of urologic disorder or disease
- History of irritative voiding symptoms
- History of pelvic irradiation
- History of chronic urinary tract infection

- History of exposure to known carcinogenic agents or chemotherapy, such as alkylating agents
- History of chronic indwelling foreign body

APPROACH TO DISCOLORED URINE THAT APPEARS AS GROSS HEMATURIA

Spin the urine by using a centrifugation device. Hematuria is present if the red color is seen in the urinary sediment. If the supernatant is red, use urinary dipstick testing on supernatant. If the dipstick test is positive for occult blood it is suggestive of myoglobin (rhabdomyolysis) or free hemoglobin caused by hemolysis. If the urine dipstick test is negative then this is suggestive of a false-positive test and is usually caused by porphyria, beets, or phenazopyridines.

Beeturia

This is the presence of red urine after ingesting beets and it is seen in 14% of beet eaters. It is caused by increased intestinal absorption of betalaine in susceptible patients. Decreased excretion of betalaine can also cause beeturia. Betalaine is protected by reducing agents, such as oxlates, and decolorized by ferric ion, hydrochloric acid, and colonic bacteria. This explains why beeturia occurs in iron deficiency anemia, achlorhydria, and oxalate ingestion (spinach, oysters, rhubarb).

Myoglobinuria

This was first described by Bywaters and Beall in 1941 during the Battle of Britain. At that time, all affected died of acute kidney injury within 1 week. Myoglobin is rapidly filtered by glomerulus and is not protein bound. It can be detected in the urine when plasma concentration is greater than 1500 ng/mL. It is caused by excessive muscle breakdown. Associated findings are elevated creatinine phosphokinase, hyperkalemia, hyperuricemia, and hyperphosphatemia with hypocalcemia.

Hemoglobinuria

Hemoglobin is poorly filtered by the glomerulus because it is a large molecule with molecular weight of 69 kDa. It is highly protein bound. March hemoglobinuria is seen with trauma to RBCs as they travel through the vasculature on dorsal aspect of feet during prolonged ambulation or marching. Urine is red or brown in color and has positive dipstick test but no RBC on urine microscopy.

SUMMARY

Hematuria is common. In many cases, particularly young adults, it is common to find hematuria that is transient and of little clinical significance. It can be microscopic or macroscopic. Microscopic hematuria is defined by presence of more than two RBCs per HPF in spun urine sediment.

Dipstick can detect one to two RBCs per HPF. Dipstick test is a good screening test, but when positive should always be followed by microscopic examination of the urine to avoid discolored urine, such as in myoglobinuria.

Determine whether hematuria is of glomerular origin as suggested by presence of proteinuria or active urine sediment (red cell cast, dysmorphic RBCs). The presence of dysmorphic RBCs, proteinuria, cellular casts, and/or renal insufficiency or any other clinical indicator suspicious for renal parenchymal disease warrants concurrent nephrologic work-up, but does not preclude the need for urologic evaluation.[29]

In patients with gross hematuria, an imaging study should be obtained. Preferred imaging modality may be multidetector CT scan with intravenous contrast. In patients with contraindications to contrast or pregnant women, consider ultrasonography as initial modality of imaging. Cystoscopy should be performed by a urologist on all patients who have evidence of gross hematuria with no evidence of bleeding.

The assessment of patients with asymptomatic microscopic hematuria should include a careful history, physical examination, and laboratory examination to rule out benign causes, such as vigorous exercise, viral illness, trauma, or recent urologic procedures.[24] Microscopic hematuria that occurs in patients who are taking anticoagulants requires urologic evaluation and nephrologic evaluation, regardless of the type or level of anticoagulation therapy.

REFERENCES

1. Froom P, Ribak J, Benbassat J. Significance of microhematuria in young adults. Br Med J (Clin Res Ed) 1984;288:20.
2. Khadra MH, Pickard RS, Charlton M, et al. A prospective analysis of 1,930 patients with hematuria to evaluate current diagnostic practice. J Urol 2000;163:524.
3. Topham PS, Harper SJ, Furness PN, et al. Glomerular disease as a cause of isolated microscopic haematuria. Q J Med 1994;87:329.
4. Messing EM, Young TB, Hunt VB, et al. The significance of asymptomatic microhematuria in men 50 or more years old: findings of a home screening study using urinary dipsticks. J Urol 1987;137:919.
5. Ritchie C, Bevan EA, Collier SJ. Importance of occult hematuria found at screening. BMJ 1986;292:681–3.
6. Denker BM, Brenner BM. Chapter on Azotemia, Urinary Abnormalities in Harrison's Principles of Internal Medicine. 17th edition. McGraw Hills Medical Publishers; 2008. p. 272–3.
7. Kallmeyer JC, Miller NM. Urinary changes in ultra- long-distance marathon runners. Nephron 1993;64:119.
8. Blacklock NJ. Bladder trauma in the long-distance runner: "10,000 metres haematuria". Br J Urol 1977;49:129.
9. Fassett RG, Owen JE, Fairley J, et al. Urinary red-cell morphology during exercise. Br Med J (Clin Res Ed) 1982;285:1455.
10. Abarbanel J, Benet AE, Lark D, et al. Sports hematuria. J Urol 1990;143(5): 887–90.
11. Smith MC, Cooke JH, Zimmerman DM et al. Asymptomatic glomerulonephritis after nonstreptococcal upper respiratory infections. Ann Intern Med 17979; 91(5):697–702.
12. Sagel I, Treser G, Ty A, et al. Occurance and nature of glomerular lesions after group A streptococci infection in childrens. Ann Intern Med 1973;79:492.
13. Britton JP, Dowell AC, Whelan P. Dipstick haematuria and bladder cancer in men over 60: results of a community study. BMJ 1989;229:1010.
14. Skinner DG, Colvin RB, Vermillion CD, et al. Diagnosis and management of renal cell carcinoma. A clinical and pathologic study of 309 cases. Cancer 1971;28: 1165–77.
15. Cokkinos P, Doulaptsis C, Chrissos D, et al. Listen to my kidney! Lancet 1944; 2009:374.
16. Górriz JL, Sancho A, Ferrer R, et al. Renal-limited polyarteritis nodosa presenting with loin pain and haematuria. Nephrol Dial Transplant 1997;12:2737.
17. Hebert LA, Betts JA, Sedmak DD, et al. Loin pain-hematuria syndrome associated with thin glomerular basement membrane disease and hemorrhage into renal tubules. Kidney Int 1996;49:168.

18. Lucas PA, Leaker BR, Murphy M, et al. Loin pain and hematuria syndrome: a somatoform disorder. QJM 1995;88:703.

19. Monnens LA. Thin glomerular basement membrane disease. Kidney Int 2001;60: 799.

20. Zhang H, Li M, Jin W, et al. The left renal entrapment syndrome: diagnosis and treatment. Ann Vasc Surg 2007;21:198.

21. Hanna HE, Santella RN, Zawada ET Jr, et al. Nutcracker syndrome: an underdiagnosed cause for hematuria? S D J Med 1997;50:429.

22. Russo D, Minutolo R, Iaccarino V, et al. Gross hematuria of uncommon origin: the nutcracker syndrome. Am J Kidney Dis 1998;32:E3.

23. Ezz el Din K, Koch WF, de Wildt MJ, et al. The predictive value of microscopic hematuria in patients with lower urinary tract symptoms and benign prostatic hyperplasia. Eur Urol 1996;30:409.

24. Mcgregor DO, Lynn KL, Bailey RR, et al. Clinical audit of the use of renal biopsy in the management of isolated microscopic hematuria. Clin Nephrol 1998;49:345.

25. Hall CL, Bradley R, Kerr A, et al. Clinical value of renal biopsy in patients with asymptomatic microscopic hematuria with and without low grade proteinuria. Clin Nephrol 2004;62:267.

26. Szeto CC, Lai FM, To KF, et al. The natural history of immunoglobulin nephropathy among patients with hematuria and minimal proteinuria. Am J Med 2001;110:434.

27. Foley SJ, Solomon LZ, Wedderburn AW, et al. A prospective study of the natural history of hematuria associated with benign prostatic hyperplasia and the effect of finasteride. J Urol 2000;163:496.

28. Eikefjord EN, Thorsen F, Rorvik J. Comparison of effective radiation doses in patients undergoing MDCT and excretory urography for acute flank pain. AJR Am J Roentgenol 2007;188:934.

29. Diagnosis, evaluation, and follow-up of asymptomatic microhematuria (AMH) in adults: American Urological Association (AUA) Guideline. Available at: http://www.auanet.org/content/media/asymptomatic_microhematuria_guideline.pdf. Approved by AUA Board of Directors 05, 2012. Accessed on June 20, 2014.

30. Grossfeld GD, Litwin MS, Wolf JS, et al. Evaluation of asymptomatic microscopic hematuria in adults: the American Urological Association best practice policy. Part I: definition, detection, prevalence, and etiology. Urology 2001;57:599.

Secondary Hypertension, Issues in Diagnosis and Treatment

Raghavesh Pullalarevu, MD[a], Ghulam Akbar, MD[a],
Geoffrey Teehan, MD, MS[b],*

KEYWORDS

- Secondary • Essential • Hyperaldosteronism • Renovascular disease • Sleep apnea
- Intrinsic kidney disease

KEY POINTS

- Resistant hypertension is more common than previously thought.
- Recent published guidelines shed new light on how to manage blood pressure and how to categorize it.
- Although essential hypertension remains the most common form of hypertension, several other entities and causes should be considered (eg, white coat hypertension, medication nonadherence, salt/alcohol abuse).
- The most common forms of resistant hypertension are obstructive sleep apnea, renal artery stenosis, primary hyperaldosteronism, and intrinsic renal disease.
- Nonpharmacologic therapies show promise but are not yet standard of care.

INTRODUCTION

Myocardial infarctions, heart failure, stroke, and noncardiac outcomes, such as end-stage renal disease, are the hallmarks of hypertension. By far the most common cardiac risk factor, hypertension outnumbers all of the remaining risk factors combined, with a prevalence of hypertension and prehypertension of 31% and 30%, respectively, in American adults.[1] Furthermore, the prevalence of hypertension with an initial episode of myocardial infarction, cerebrovascular disease, and congestive heart failure is 69%, 77%, and 74%, respectively.[2] Its economic impact in the United States is staggering, costing $47.5 billion for treatment and $3.5 billion in lost productivity annually.[3]

[a] Division of Nephrology, Department of Medicine, Lankenau Medical Center, 100 E Lancaster Ave, Wynnewood, PA 19096, USA; [b] Division of Nephrology, Department of Medicine, Lankenau Institute of Medical Research, Lankenau Medical Center, 100 E Lancaster Ave, Wynnewood, PA 19096, USA
* Corresponding author.
E-mail address: gteehan@comcast.net

Prim Care Clin Office Pract 41 (2014) 749–764
http://dx.doi.org/10.1016/j.pop.2014.08.001   **primarycare.theclinics.com**

The definition of hypertension has undergone some modification in the wake of the newly reported findings of the Eighth Joint National Committee (JNC 8) released in late 2013, and expands on the definitions established in the JNC 7. The European Society of Hypertension (ESH) and the European Society of Cardiology (ESC) add to this by assigning a risk class to various levels of blood pressure (BP) (**Tables 1** and **2**). These updated hypertensive standards impact the interpretation of secondary hypertension (SH).[4–6]

INCIDENCE/PREVALENCE

The incidence of SH is unknown but may be as high as 10% in newly diagnosed hypertensive patients. Persell[7] estimates the prevalence to be 12.8% among those treated with antihypertensive medications. Furthermore, inadequate treatment or poor BP control from nonadherence with both pharmacologic and nonpharmacologic therapy may lead to overdiagnosing resistant hypertension.[8]

DISEASE DESCRIPTIONS

Several defined forms of hypertension exist:

- Essential (primary) hypertension (EH): most common. Lacks a specific known causative medical condition or disease. Genetics, poor diet, lack of exercise, and obesity are usual aggravating factors.[9]
- White coat hypertension (isolated clinic or office hypertension): office BP readings usually greater than 140/90 mm Hg and reliable out-of-office readings that are routinely less than 140/90 mm Hg.[10]
- Masked hypertension: office BP readings less than 140/90 mm Hg but ambulatory or home BP readings in the hypertensive range.[11]
- Pseudohypertension: suggested when radial pulse remains palpable despite occlusion of the brachial artery by the cuff (Osler maneuver).[12]
- Resistant hypertension: BP 140/90 mm Hg or greater despite adherence to treatment with full doses of at least 3 antihypertensive medications, including a diuretic.[4]
- Refractory hypertension: similar to resistant hypertension but requires 4 drugs to meet the criteria, and patients generally respond poorly to mineralocorticoid antagonists.[13]

Table 1
JNC 7 definitions

BP (mm Hg)	Category
<120/<80	Normal
SBP, 120–139 or DBP, 80–89	Prehypertension
SBP, 140–159 or DBP, 90–99	Stage I hypertension
SBP ≥160, DBP ≥100	Stage II hypertension

Abbreviations: DBP, diastolic blood pressure; SBP, systolic blood pressure.
Data from Chobanian AV, Bakris GL, Black HR, et al, National Heart, Lung, and Blood Institute Joint National Committee on Prevention, Detection, Evaluation, and Treatment of High Blood Pressure, National High Blood Pressure Education Program Coordinating Committee. The seventh report of the Joint National Committee on Prevention, Detection, Evaluation, and Treatment of High Blood Pressure: the JNC 7 report. JAMA 2003;289(19):2560–72.

Table 2
European Society of Hypertension and the European Society of Cardiology hypertension framework

Risk Category	High Normal: SBP, 130–139 mm Hg or DBP, 85–89 mm Hg	Grade I HTN: SBP, 140–159 mm Hg or DBP, 90–99 mm Hg	Grade 2 HTN: SBP, 160–179 mm Hg or DBP, 100–109 mm Hg	Grade 3 HTN: SBP ≥180 mm Hg or DBP ≥110 mm Hg
No RFs		Low risk	Moderate risk	High risk
1–2 RFs	Low risk	Moderate risk	Moderate to high risk	High risk
≥3 RFs	Low to moderate risk	Moderate to high risk	High risk	High risk
OD, CKD stage III, or diabetes	Moderate to high risk	High risk	High risk	High risk to very high risk
Symptomatic CVD, CKD ≥ stage IV, or patients with diabetes with OD/RF	Very high risk	Very high risk	Very high risk	Very high risk

Abbreviations: CKD, chronic kidney disease; CVD, cardiovascular disease; DBP, diastolic blood pressure; HTN, hypertension; OD, organ damage; RF, risk factor; SBP, systolic blood pressure.

Adapted from Mancia G, Fagard R, Narkiewicz K, et al. 2013 ESH/ESC guidelines for the management of arterial hypertension: the Task Force for the Management of Arterial Hypertension of the European Society of Hypertension (ESH) and of the European Society of Cardiology (ESC). Eur Heart J 2013;34(28):2159–219.

SECONDARY HYPERTENSION

SH often implies a correctable form of hypertension, may be diagnosed in a subset of patients with nonessential hypertension, and is often suspected when certain clues prompt a more extensive evaluation of the causes of the hypertension. In the evolution of an SH workup, however, often several correctable/modifiable factors are uncovered.[1] This article focuses on the definition, differential diagnosis, epidemiology, and treatment of SH.

RISK FACTORS

Box 1 lists common issues facing the clinician in dealing with difficult-to-control hypertension, most notably the high sodium diet. Pimenta and colleagues[14] studied 12 patients with hypertension and showed that a low versus high sodium diet (after a washout period) resulted in a BP decrease of 23/9 mm Hg on routine cuff measurement and 20/10 on ambulatory BP monitoring (ABPM). The use of ABPM to diagnose white coat hypertension is gaining favor as reimbursement for testing is starting to occur. Other common causes include nonsteroidal use, sedentary lifestyle, and excessive alcohol consumption.[1]

After potentially correctable issues are addressed, other symptoms that may indicate a diagnosis SH include[21]:

- An acute increase in previously well-controlled BP
- Malignant or accelerated hypertension (with signs of end-organ damage)
- Age less than 30 years

Box 1
Modifiable risk factors for hypertension

Lifestyle modifications include

1. Exercise: advised most days of the week for at least 30–45 minutes.[1]

2. Dietary sodium intake less than 2.3 g/d: may lower the systolic BP (SBP)/diastolic BP (DBP) by 4.8/2.5 mm Hg.[15]

3. Weight loss: for every 1 kg decrease in weight, DBP decreases by 0.5–2.0 mm Hg.[16]

4. DASH (Dietary Approaches to Stop Hypertension); promotes more fruits, vegetables, and low-fat dairy products (reduced saturated and total fat); reduces BP by 5.5/3.0 mm Hg.[17]

5. Vitamin D treatment: for patients with low or low-normal vitamin D levels or people at risk; vitamin D deficiency is associated with incident hypertension in winter months especially.[18]

6. Moderation of alcohol intake: $\leq$2 alcohol-containing drinks in women and $\leq$3 in men may significantly reduce mean BP (3.3/2.0 mm Hg).[19]

7. Avoid sympathomimetics (ephedra, phenylephrine, cocaine, amphetamines, herbal supplements [ginseng, yohimbine], anabolic steroids, appetite suppressants, nonsteroidal anti-inflammatory drugs, and erythropoietin).[20]

- Patient is nonobese, non-Black; particularly those in whom onset precedes puberty
- Abnormal laboratory values and imaging results

Recognizing that most hypertension diagnosed in the office/clinical setting represents EH, using these clues to isolate particular patients who may benefit from a more exhaustive workup could limit unnecessary testing. Furthermore, although the differential diagnosis of SH is sufficiently broad, a few conditions predominate and limit the extent of any given workup.

DISEASE STATES AND WORKUP

Table 3 lists the causes of SH. Renovascular disease, intrinsic renal disease, primary hyperaldosteronism, and obstructive sleep apnea represent the most common causes of SH.[22]

RENOVASCULAR HYPERTENSION

Renovascular hypertension is suspected when the following are noted[26,27]:

- Severe or refractory hypertension
- Unexplained acute increase in serum creatinine of more than 30% after initiating a renin-angiotensin system inhibitor (ACEI) or angiotensin receptor blocker (ARB), also known as *ischemic nephropathy.*
- Uncontrolled hypertension in a patient with diffuse atherosclerosis
- Unexplained renal asymmetry (ie, a unilateral small kidney)
- Recurrent episodes of flash pulmonary edema
- Renal dysfunction following initiation of a diuretic
- Abdominal bruit
- Uncontrolled hypertension in younger-aged woman or older man with severe atherosclerotic disease
- Unprovoked hypokalemia

Renovascular hypertension classically manifests as renal artery stenosis (RAS) or fibromuscular dysplasia. The former occurs in older patients and those with peripheral arterial disease, hyperlipidemia, and a previous history of tobacco use, whereas the latter more commonly occurs in younger women with new onset hypertension. **Table 4** outlines these differences.

The diagnosis is usually made in the setting of malignant hypertension and occasionally the finding of an abdominal bruit, which prompts some form of imaging. A renal duplex ultrasound lacks the sensitivity and specificity of computed tomography (CT) or MR angiography, but avoids the pitfalls of radiocontrast nephropathy in the former and nephrogenic systemic fibrosis in the latter. Therapy in both cases is aimed at primarily lowering BP, but interventional approaches differ significantly. In fibromuscular dysplasia, percutaneous transluminal angioplasty (PTLA) and stenting is associated with cure of hypertension in 22% to 59% of patients, and improved BP in 22% to 74%.[26] Several randomized, controlled, clinical trials have found no benefit for PTLA/stenting in RAS. The STAR, ASTRAL, and CORAL trials showed no benefit and have led to the collective conclusion that treatment of RAS should be directed at controlling BP and hyperlipidemia, and reducing risk of progressive narrowing of the renal arteries through antiplatelet therapy, even though RAS is severely occlusive.[33–35]

Because the diseases are associated with elevated plasma renin activity and serum aldosterone levels, ACEI and ARB may be reasonable choices, but if the stenoses are critical, this may lead to ischemic nephropathy. Renal chemistries should be checked within 1 to 2 weeks of initiating therapy, and starting at a low dose may be helpful.[33]

INTRINSIC RENAL DISEASE

The diagnosis is usually intuitive and based on abnormal serum creatinine and blood urea nitrogen levels. The proximate cause of kidney disease can be informative. Hypertension can occur as a natural consequence of advancing chronic kidney disease (CKD) by virtue of fewer nephrons available to process salt and water. The urinalysis may be bland. Acute glomerulonephritis, however, can manifest with new-onset, difficult-to-control hypertension but can be associated with vastly different urinary findings, and classically with hematuria and red blood cell casts. Adult polycystic kidney disease can cause SH. Kidney tumors such as renal cell carcinoma, nephroblastoma, and renin-producing tumors vasculitis involving renal vasculature such polyarteritis nodosa and chronic pyelonephritis can also cause SH. In most cases a referral to a nephrologist is warranted. The goal of therapy in intrinsic kidney disease is to reduce the BP, reduce the risk of the cardiovascular events, and halt or slow the progression of kidney disease. The therapy of hypertension may then depend on the cause.[36,37]

In hypertension associated with CKD (intrinsic renal disease), first-line therapy is an ACEI or ARB, particularly if proteinuria/albuminuria is present.[5] Activation of the renin angiotensin-aldosterone system underlies the use of ACEIs or ARBs as the drugs of choice. In any form of intrinsic kidney disease, intraglomerular pressure is elevated, leading to glomerular hypertension and hyperfiltration injury. ACEIs or ARBs reduce intraglomerular pressure and thereby help to preserve renal function, although often with a small increase in the measured serum creatinine level.[38] Autoregulation largely compensates for this decline in glomerular filtration rate (GFR), but this effect can be marked in patients with bilateral renal artery stenosis (or unilateral with solitary kidney function), volume-depleted states, hypertensive nephrosclerosis, and vasculitis, such as polyarteritis nodosa. ACEI/ARB-induced reduction in GFR usually occurs within a few days after initiation therapy and is almost always reversible with cessation of

Table 3
Causes of secondary hypertension

Cause	Signs & Symptoms	Diagnostic Tests/Findings	Treatment
Primary aldosteronism[23]	Fatigue, hypokalemia, metabolic alkalosis, hypernatremia	High aldosterone/renin ratio (>20) or aldosterone level >15 ng/dL	Aldosterone antagonists, ACEI or ARB as adjuvant therapy Surgery for adenoma
Intrinsic renal disease[5]	Fatigue, nocturia, frothy urine, hematuria	Urinalysis with RBC/WBC casts Elevated serum creatinine level	ACEI or ARB first-line, thiazide diuretic, loop diuretic (GFR <30 mL/min), calcium channel blocker
Sleep apnea syndrome[24]	Fatigue, obesity, daytime somnolence, poor sleep quality, snoring	Polysomnography	Weight loss, nocturnal CPAP
Pheochromocytoma[25]	Interval episodes of hypertension, with flushing, diaphoresis, headaches	Elevated urine norepinephrine (>80 mcg/24 h), VMA (>5 mg/24 h), plasma metanephrines CT/MRI of abdomen	α-blocker and, if needed, β-blocker; β-blockers not as sole therapy Surgical excision
Renal artery disease[26,27]	Young women with abdominal bruit Older patients with accelerated hypertension, tobacco abuse, peripheral arterial disease	Increased serum creatinine level with ACEI/ARB (>30%), MR angiography, disparity in kidney size on duplex ultrasound	Angioplasty/stent not superior to medical management[14] Avoid ACEI/ARB Use calcium channel blockers, diuretics, aldosterone antagonists

Condition	Clinical features	Diagnosis	Treatment
Hypothyroidism & hyperthyroidism[28]	Fatigue, bradycardia, weight gain, abnormal menstrual cycle, increased DBP (hypothyroidism), weight loss & anxiety, tachycardia, increased SBP (hyperthyroidism)	TSH, free T4	Thyroid replacement therapy, surgery
Cushing syndrome[29]	Obesity, abnormal menstrual cycle, abdominal striae, hyperglycemia, muscle weakness, skin ecchymoses	Increased urine cortisol level (>55 mcg/24 h), positive DST, reduced renin & aldosterone levels, imaging on CT/MRI	Surgery
Coarctation of aorta[30]	Brachial-femoral delay in pulse, hypertension on upper extremities, low or normal blood pressure in lower extremities, to-and-fro machinery murmur	Two-dimensional echocardiography, chest CT & MRI	Surgery, angioplasty
Oral contraceptive pills (OCP)[6]	Fatigue, headaches	Onset of hypertension with OCP, weight gain	Stop OCP
Liddle syndrome[31]	Fatigue, headaches, severe hypertension, young age, hypokalemia,	Reduced plasma renin & aldosterone levels, renal potassium wasting	Salt restriction, amiloride
Primary hyperparathyroidism[32]	Abdominal pain, bone pain, kidney stones and psychiatric issues	Elevated iPTH level, increased serum calcium level, hypophosphatemia, anemia	Surgery, bisphosphonates, calcimimetics

Abbreviations: ACEI, angiotensin converting enzyme inhibitor; ARB, angiotensin receptor blocker; CPAP, continuous positive airway pressure; DBP, diastolic blood pressure; DST, dexamethasone suppression test; iPTH, intact parathyroid hormone; RBC, red blood cell; SBP, systolic blood pressure; WBC, white blood cell.

Table 4
Fibromuscular dysplasia and renal artery stenosis: comparison

	Fibromuscular Dysplasia	Renal Artery Stenosis
Age of onset	Younger	Older
Location of lesion	Middle to distal two-thirds of renal artery	Ostial
Response to revascularization	Cures hypertension in 22%–59% of patients Improves hypertension in 22%–74% of patients	Poor; associated with risk of contrast nephropathy, atheroembolic disease, dissection
Medical therapy to control BP	ACEI/ARB first-line (not n pregnant patients); thiazide diuretic second-line	ACEI/ARB (may cause ischemic nephropathy)
Goals of therapy	BP control	BP control; lipid-lowering and antiplatelet therapy
Radiographic diagnosis	Renal artery duplex, CT/MR angiography	Renal artery duplex, CT/MR angiography

Data from Slovut DP, Olin JW. Fibromuscular dysplasia. N Engl J Med 2004;350:1862.

drug. A less than 30% increase in serum creatinine concentration is considered acceptable after administration of ACEI/ARBs, and follow-up blood tests within 1 to 2 weeks are recommended.[39]

In acute glomerulonephritis, treating hypertension may still respond to ACEI/ARB, particularly because these diseases typically manifest proteinuria, but the underlying form of glomerulonephritis will also dictate therapy, which could include pulsed steroids, immunosuppressants, monoclonal antibodies, or chemotherapy.

KIDNEY TRANSPLANT

Hypertension, when defined as a BP greater than 140/90 mm Hg, may be present in 50% to 80% of kidney transplant recipients. Its presence is associated with worse long-term graft outcome, including graft loss. Calcineurin inhibitors and steroids contribute to a secondary hypertension-like effect by causing vasoconstriction and salt retention, with weight gain and a mineralocorticoid effect, respectively.[4,40,41]

PRIMARY HYPERALDOSTERONISM

Increased autonomous production of the mineralocorticoid aldosterone by the adrenal gland, combined with suppressed renin secretion by the kidneys, are the hallmarks of primary hyperaldosteronism (PHA). It may be caused by an adrenal adenoma, unilateral or bilateral adrenal hyperplasia, or, rarely, an adrenocortical carcinoma. Major clues to consider the diagnosis of PHA include resistant hypertension in a patient with hypokalemia, metabolic alkalosis, and mild hypernatremia. **Box 2** lists additional common clues to the diagnosis of PHA. Although hypokalemia is considered the hallmark feature of PHA, Mulatero and colleagues[42] showed that almost 60% of patients with PHA were normokalemic.

Screening for PHA begins by testing an early morning blood sample for serum aldosterone, plasma renin activity (PRA), and the associated aldosterone-to-renin ratio (ARR). PRA is characteristically very low or undetectable in PHA. On the other hand, it is increased in patients with hypokalemia and hypertension who also have

---

Box 2
Screening for PHA

In 2008, The Endocrine Society recommended that the following clinical features prompt consideration of screening for PHA based on the ratio of plasma aldosterone concentration to plasma renin activity:

- Hypertension and spontaneous or low-dose diuretic-induced hypokalemia

- Severe hypertension (>160 mm Hg systolic or >100 mm Hg diastolic) or drug-resistant hypertension (defined as suboptimally controlled hypertension on a 3-drug program that includes an adrenergic inhibitor, vasodilator, and diuretic)

- Hypertension with adrenal incidentaloma

- Hypertension and a family history of early-onset hypertension or cerebrovascular accident at a young age (<40 years)

- All hypertensive first-degree relatives of patients with primary aldosteronism

Data from Funder JW, Carey RM, Fardella C, et al. Case detection, diagnosis, and treatment of patients with primary aldosteronism: an Endocrine Society clinical practice guideline. J Clin Endocrinol Metab 2008;93(9):3266.

---

renovascular disease, a renin-secreting tumor, malignant hypertension, or coarctation of the aorta, or who are undergoing concomitant diuretic therapy. This test is more sensitive than plasma aldosterone alone and more specific than an isolated PRA level. An ARR greater than 20 suggests a diagnosis of PHA (sensitivity, 78%–89%; specificity, 71%–83%).[43]

Considerable debate exists about whether to stop all antihypertensives to perform assays of renin and aldosterone. **Table 5** outlines the disease states associated with various levels of PRA and serum aldosterone. Older guidelines suggested stopping all drugs for up to 6 weeks to get a "pure" reading on renin and aldosterone, but this is associated with a real risk of causing problems such as hypertensive emergency,

---

Table 5
Utility of plasma aldosterone and renin level and ratios in hypertension with/without hypokalemia and metabolic alkalosis

Laboratory Data	Associated Clinical Conditions
High renin and high aldosterone	Secondary hyperaldosteronism • Renovascular hypertension • Renin-secreting tumor • Diuretic use • Malignant hypertension • Coarctation of aorta
Low renin, high aldosterone	Primary hyperaldosteronism
Low renin, low aldosterone	Increased nonaldosterone mineralocorticoid activity • Congenital adrenal hyperplasia • Cushing syndrome • Liddle syndrome • Licorice root ingestion • Deoxycorticosterone-producing adrenal tumors

Data from McKenna TJ, Sequeira SJ, Heffernan A, et al. Diagnosis under random conditions of all disorders of the renin-angiotensin-aldosterone axis, including primary hyperaldosteronism. J Clin Endocrinol Metab 1991;73:952.

arrhythmia, or heart failure during this extended drug-free period. Some authors recommend substituting agents like slow-acting verapamil, hydralazine, or prazosin, which have little if any effect on these hormones, but their use must be weighed against the potential for harm in the patient in question. Further, this forces patients to purchase new BP agents and can be cumbersome. β-blockers, clonidine, and α-methyldopa reduce renin levels, whereas diuretics, ACEIs, and dihydropyridine calcium channel blockers increase renin levels. The authors advocate stopping miner-alocorticoid receptor antagonists because they will alter the interpretation of aldoste-rone level, but to continue remaining agents.[44]

A positive screening test of ARR is confirmed by an aldosterone suppression test to confirm nonsuppressibility. This suppression is usually accomplished by oral or intra-venous salt loading. Captopril challenge or a fludrocortisone suppression test are additional options to confirm the positive findings of elevated ARR.[45]

In suspected PHA, a radiographic diagnosis is in order. Adrenal CT scan is the initial imaging modality of choice to distinguish among the causes of PHA (aldo-sterone-producing adenoma, unilateral/bilateral adrenal hyperplasia, and adrenal carcinoma). In special circumstances, adrenal vein sampling can be performed by an experienced interventional radiologist to diagnose unilateral adrenal hyperplasia.[46]

Adrenal adenomas are typically managed successfully by surgical resection. Sur-gical resection can be considered in people with unilateral adrenal hyperplasia, but bilateral adrenal hyperplasia is best managed medically with MR angiography.[47,48]

OBSTRUCTIVE SLEEP APNEA

Obstructive sleep apnea (OSA) classically occurs in obese individuals and those with advanced CKD. Resistant hypertension is a common and emerging feature, and its severity directly correlates with the apnea.[49,50] OSA is an independent risk factor for the development of hypertension and predicts resistance to antihypertensive therapy. Response to continuous positive airway pressure (CPAP) is variable. Marin and colleagues,[51] showed that CPAP treatment can reduce the incidence of new-onset hy-pertension in people with OSA. Barbé and colleagues,[52] however, failed to confirm this preventive role. A review of meta-analyses showed that CPAP therapy in OSA has a small but statistically significant effect on BP reduction.[53]

CUSHING SYNDROME

Cushing syndrome is often diagnosed clinically when patients present with cushingoid facies, proximal muscle weakness, central obesity, and ecchymoses. In other cases, as part of a resistant hypertension workup, imaging will disclose an adrenal incidenta-loma or small cell lung cancer (paraneoplastic-ectopic adrenocorticotropic hormone secretion). Alternatively, patients receiving chronic glucocorticoids may develop resistant hypertension. Although the reported incidence of hypertension in Cushing syndrome ranges from 74% to 87%, only a minority of these cases is SH. The diag-nosis can be made by collecting a 24-hour urine sample and showing a urine cortisol level greater than 55 mcg. A positive dexamethasone suppression test (failure to sup-press cortisol to less than 3 mcg after administration of 1 mg of dexamethasone) and CT or MRI studies can help secure the diagnosis. Although surgical treatment is the best option, medical management is performed until surgery, and includes (1) adrenal enzyme inhibitors, such as ketoconazole, etomidate, and metapyrone; (2) adrenolytic agents, such as mitotane; and (3) dopamine agonists, such as cabergoline and pasireotide.[54–56]

COARCTATION OF THE AORTA

Aortic coarctation usually manifests in youth and accounts for less than 1% of all causes of hypertension.[2] The 2013 ESH/ESC suggests assessing for coarctation of the aorta as part of the workup for patients with congenital heart diseases and SH through palpating brachial and femoral arteries simultaneously. Classic findings include hypertension in upper extremities and hypotension in lower extremities, along with a brachial-femoral pulse delay and a systolic-diastolic ("to-and-fro") murmur heard on the chest. Management options include surgery, balloon angioplasty, and stent placement.[30]

ORAL CONTRACEPTIVE PILLS

Oral contraceptive pill (OCP) use may be associated with a BP increase of 3 to 6/2 to 5 mm Hg, with 5% of patients developing frank hypertension. Malignant hypertension has also been reported. Hypertensive effects are thought to be dose-dependent, and current-day OCPs have very low doses of estrogen and progesterone compared with those in the past. However, a 1.8% and 1.2% relative risk for hypertension still exists for current and prior users of low-dosed OCPs. BP normalizes in these patients after cessation of therapy.[57,58]

LIDDLE SYNDROME

Liddle syndrome is a rare autosomal dominant disease that usually manifests in childhood. Enhanced activity of sodium channels in the distal tubules of the kidney leads to increased sodium water absorption, causing volume overload and hypertension. A hypokalemic metabolic alkalosis and suppressed plasma renin and aldosterone levels are observed. Potassium-sparing diuretics, particularly amiloride and triamterene, are the drugs of choice.[31]

PRIMARY HYPERPARATHYROIDISM

Primary hyperparathyroidism is associated with not only hypertension but also left ventricular hypertrophy and diastolic dysfunction. Although no comprehensive explanation exists for this, Walker and colleagues[32] found increased carotid intima-media thickness and increased carotid vascular and aortic stiffness in patients with primary hyperparathyroidism, suggesting that vessel stiffness may be causative. A nuclear scan can diagnose a parathyroid adenoma, and surgical resection or cinacalcet are the available treatment options.[59]

HYPOTHYROIDISM/HYPERTHYROIDISM

Hypothyroidism is an unusual cause of SH and is believed to produce an increase in peripheral vascular resistance, and may exacerbate preexisting hypertension. Isolated systolic hypertension has been observed in hyperthyroidism. Treatment involves replacing lost hormone production, surgery to remove overactive tissue, or radioactive therapies.[28,60]

PHEOCHROMOCYTOMA

Pheochromocytomas, which are usually adrenal-based tumors, should be suspected in patients with a history of paroxysmal hypertension, often complicated by palpitations, sweating, and headache ("classic triad"). The hypertension is labile and resistant. It can be associated with multiple endocrine neoplasia 2. An adrenal incidentaloma with drug-resistant hypertension should cause suspicion for pheochromocytoma. The true incidence is unknown but is estimated to account for 0.2% of patients with hypertension.[61] The "rule of 10s" applies to pheochromocytoma: 10% are malignant, 10% are bilateral, and 10% are extra-adrenal.

The diagnosis requires a 24-hour urine collection for metanephrines, followed by a CT scan or MRI of abdomen/adrenal glands. Urine metanephrine levels should be drawn if pretest probability is very high, because the condition is rare. These have a high sensitivity and specificity (98% for each). Plasma metanephrine levels can help solidify the diagnosis.[62] A metaiodobenzylguanidine scintigraphy scan or octreoscan can be performed if initial imaging results are negative but strong clinical suspicion persists.[63] Surgery is the treatment of choice. Preoperative α-blockade (phenoxybenzamine) initially, followed by β-blockers, is the medical treatment of choice.[61]

NEW DIRECTIONS: EXPERIMENTAL THERAPIES FOR RESISTANT HYPERTENSION
Renal Denervation

Renal denervation involves radiofrequency ablation of renal sympathetic nerves using a angiographically directed catheter. Symplicity HTN-2, a randomized trial performed largely in European centers, studied the effect of renal denervation in 106 patients with resistant hypertension and reported a significant BP reduction from 178/97 to 143/85 mm Hg compared with no reduction in BP in people maintained on medical therapy.[64] The Symplicity HTN-3 trial, which followed a similar protocol in United States–based centers, enrolled 530 patients and was terminated (results pending), suggesting that the effect seen in Symplicity HTN-2 was not duplicated. For now, renal denervation is not approved by the U.S. Food and Drug Administration and remains experimental.

ELECTRICAL STIMULATION OF CAROTID SINUS BARORECEPTORS

Carotid sinus baroreceptor stimulation using an implanted electrical device leads to a baroreflex system–mediated decrease in BP. Although initial studies have been promising, it is a cumbersome and invasive therapy. The Rheos Pivotal Trial randomized 265 patients with resistant hypertension to use the device (turn it on) or not use the device (leave it off). At 6 months, no significant differences in BP reduction were seen, although patients randomized to active therapy were significantly more likely to achieve a systolic BP less than 140 mm Hg. At 1 month, 35% of patients experienced a serious procedure-related adverse event. Larger studies are needed to confirm its long-term efficacy and determine the procedure-related complications.[65]

SUMMARY

Resistant hypertension is more common than once thought. The most recent published guidelines on BP management shed new light on how to manage BP and how to categorize it. Although EH remains the most common form of hypertension, several other entities and causes should be considered (eg, white coat hypertension, medication nonadherence, salt/alcohol abuse). The most common forms of resistant hypertension are OSA, renal artery stenosis, primary hyperaldosteronism, and intrinsic renal disease. After these, a more dedicated workup will depend on laboratory and imaging findings. Nonpharmacologic therapies show promise but are not yet standard of care.

REFERENCES

1. Calhoun DA, Jones D, Textor S, et al. Resistant hypertension: diagnosis, evaluation and treatment: a scientific statement from the American Heart Association Professional Education Committee of the Council for High Blood Pressure Research. Circulation 2008;117:e510.
2. Roger VL, Go AS, Lloyd-Jones DM, et al. Heart disease and stroke statistics—2012 update: a report from the American Heart Association. Circulation 2012;125(1):e2–220.
3. Heidenreich PA, Trogdon JG, Khavjou OA, et al. Forecasting the future of cardiovascular disease in the United States: a policy statement from the American Heart Association. Circulation 2011;123(8):933–44.
4. Chobanian AV, Bakris GL, Black HR, et al, National Heart, Lung, and Blood Institute Joint National Committee on Prevention, Detection, Evaluation, and Treatment of High Blood Pressure, National High Blood Pressure Education Program Coordinating Committee. The seventh report of the Joint National Committee on Prevention, Detection, Evaluation, and Treatment of High Blood Pressure: the JNC 7 report. JAMA 2003;289(19):2560–72.
5. James P, Oparil S, Carter BL, et al. 2014 Evidenced-based guideline for the management of high blood pressure in adults. Report from the panel members are pointed to the Eighth Joint National Committee (JNC 8). JAMA 2014;311(5):507–20.
6. Mancia G, Fagard R, Narkiewicz K, et al. 2013 ESH/ESC guidelines for the management of arterial hypertension: the Task Force for the Management of Arterial Hypertension of the European Society of Hypertension (ESH) and of the European Society of Cardiology (ESC). Eur Heart J 2013;34(28):2159–219.
7. Persell SD. Prevalence of resistant hypertension in the United States, 2003-2008. Hypertension 2011;57(6):1076.
8. de la Sierra A, Segura J, Banegas JR, et al. Clinical features of 8295 patients with resistant hypertension classified on the basis of ambulatory blood pressure monitoring. Hypertension 2011;57:898.
9. Centers for Disease Control and Prevention (CDC). Vital signs: prevalence, treatment, and control of hypertension—United States, 1999-2002 and 2005-2008. MMWR Morb Mortal Wkly Rep 2011;60(4):103–8.
10. Myers MG. A proposed algorithm for diagnosing hypertension using automated office blood pressure measurement. J Hypertens 2010;28:703.
11. Papadopoulos DP, Makris TK. Masked hypertension definition, impact, outcomes: a critical review. J Clin Hypertens (Greenwich) 2007;9(12):956–63.
12. Messerli FH, Ventura HO, Amodeo C. Osler's maneuver and pseudo-hypertension. N Engl J Med 1985;312:1548–51.
13. Acelajado MC, Pisoni R, Dudenbostel T, et al. Refractory hypertension: definition, prevalence, and patient characteristics. J Clin Hypertens (Greenwich) 2012;14:7.
14. Pimenta E, Gaddam KK, Oparil S, et al. Effects of dietary sodium reduction on blood pressure and subjects with resistant hypertension: results from a randomized trial. Hypertension 2009;54:475.
15. Appel LJ. Dietary approaches to prevent and treat hypertension: a scientific statement from the American Heart Association. Hypertension 2006;47(2):296.
16. Stevens VJ. Weight loss intervention in phase 1 of the Trials of Hypertension Prevention. The TOHP Collaborative Research Group. Arch Intern Med 1993;153(7):849.
17. Appel LJ. A clinical trial of the effects of dietary patterns on blood pressure. DASH Collaborative Research Group. N Engl J Med 1997;336(16):1117.

18. Larsen T. Effect of cholecalciferol supplementation during winter months in patients with hypertension: a randomized, placebo-controlled trial. Am J Hypertens 2012;25(11):1215–22.

19. Xin X. Effects of alcohol reduction on blood pressure: a meta-analysis of randomized controlled trials. Hypertension 2001;38(5):1112.

20. Mancia G, De Backer G, Dominiczak A, et al. 2007 guidelines for the management of arterial hypertension: the task force for the management of arterial hypertension of the European Society of Hypertension (ESH) and of the European Society Cardiology (ESC). J Hypertens 2007;25:1105.

21. Lewin A, Blaufox MD, Castle H, et al. Apparent prevalence of curable hypertension in the Hypertension Detection and Follow-up Program. Arch Intern Med 1985;145:424.

22. Goodfriend TL, Calhoun DA. Resistant hypertension, obesity, sleep apnea, and aldosterone: theory and therapy. Hypertension 2004;43:518.

23. Douma S, Petidis K, Doumas M, et al. Prevalence of primary hyperaldosteronism in resistant hypertension: a retrospective observational study. Lancet 2008;371:1921.

24. Somers VK, White DP, Amin R, et al. Sleep apnea and cardiovascular disease: an American Heart Association/American College of Cardiology Foundation Scientific Statement from the American Council on Clinical Cardiology, Stroke Council, and Council on Cardiovascular Nursing. J Am Coll Cardiol 2008;52:686.

25. Beard CM, Sheps SG, Kurland LT, et al. Occurrence of pheochromocytoma in Rochester, Minnesota, 1950 through 1979. Mayo Clin Proc 1983;58(12):802.

26. Slovut DP, Olin JW. Fibromuscular dysplasia. N Engl J Med 2004;350:1862.

27. Tullis MJ, Caps MT, Zierler RE, et al. Blood pressure, antihypertensive medication, and atherosclerotic renal artery stenosis. Am J Kidney Dis 1999;33:675.

28. Streeten DH, Anderson GH Jr, Howland T, et al. Effects of thyroid function on blood pressure. Recognition of hypothyroid hypertension. Hypertension 1988;11:78.

29. Orth DN. Cushing's syndrome. N Engl J Med 1995;332:791.

30. Warnes CA, Williams RG, Bashore TM, et al. ACC/AHA 2008 Guidelines for the Management of Adults with Congenital Heart Disease: a report of the American College of Cardiology/American Heart Association Task Force on Practice Guidelines. Circulation 2008;118:e714.

31. Palmer BF, Alpern RJ. Liddle's syndrome. Am J Med 1998;104:301.

32. Lind L, Jacobsson S, Palmér M, et al. Cardiovascular risk factors in primary hyperparathyroidism: a 15 year follow-up of operated and unoperated cases. J Intern Med 1991;230:29.

33. Bax L, Woittiez AJ, Kouwenberg HJ, et al. Stent placement in patients with atherosclerotic renal artery stenosis and impaired renal function: a randomized trial. Ann Intern Med 2009;150:840.

34. The ASTRAL Investigators. Revascularization versus medical therapy for renal-artery stenosis. N Engl J Med 2009;361:1953.

35. Cooper C, Murphy TP, Cutlip DE, et al. Stenting and medical therapy for atherosclerotic renal-artery stenosis. N Engl J Med 2014;370:13.

36. Bakris GL, Ritz E. The message for World Kidney Day 2009: hypertension and kidney disease: a marriage that should be prevented. Kidney Int 2009;75:449.

37. Hall JE, Guyton AC, Jackson TE, et al. Control of glomerular filtration rate by renin-angiotensin system. Am J Physiol 1977;233(5):F366.

38. Hollenberg NK, Swartz SL, Passan DR, et al. Filtration rate after converting-enzyme inhibition in essential hypertension. N Engl J Med 1979;301(1):9.

39. Toto RD, Mitchell HC, Lee HC, et al. Reversible renal insufficiency due to angiotensin converting enzyme inhibitors in hypertensive nephrosclerosis. Ann Intern Med 1991;115(7):513.
40. Kasiske BL, Anjum S, Shah R, et al. Hypertension after kidney transplantation. Am J Kidney Dis 2004;43:1071.
41. Opelz G, Wujciak T, Ritz E. Association of chronic kidney graft failure with recipient blood pressure. Collaborative Transplant Study. Kidney Int 1998;53:217.
42. Mulatero P, Stowasser M, Loh KC, et al. Increased diagnosis of primary aldosteronism, including surgically correctable forms, in centers from five continents. J Clin Endocrinol Metab 2004;89(3):1045.
43. Nishizaka MK, Pratt-Ubunama M, Zaman MA, et al. Validity of plasma aldosterone to renin activity ratio in African American and white subjects with resistant hypertension. Am J Hypertens 2005;18:805–12.
44. Gallay BJ, Ahmad S, Xu L, et al. Screening for primary aldosteronism without discontinuing hypertensive medications: plasma aldosterone-renin ratio. Am J Kidney Dis 2001;37(4):699.
45. Carey RM, Fardella C, Gomez-Sanchez CE, et al. Case detection, diagnosis, and treatment of patients with primary aldosteronism: an Endocrine Society clinical practice guideline. J Clin Endocrinol Metab 2008;93(9):3266.
46. Young WF, Stanson AW, Thompson GB, et al. Role for adrenal venous sampling in primary aldosteronism. Surgery 2004;136(6):1227.
47. Milsom SR, Espiner EA, Nicholls MG, et al. The blood pressure response to unilateral adrenalectomy in primary aldosteronism. Q J Med 1986;61(236):1141.
48. Lim PO, Young WF, MacDonald TM. A review of the medical treatment of primary aldosteronism. J Hypertens 2001;19(3):353.
49. Gonçalves SC, Martinez D, Gus M, et al. Obstructive sleep apnea and resistant hypertension: a case-control study. Chest 2007;132(6):1858.
50. Pedrosa RP, Drager LF, Gonzaga CC, et al. Obstructive sleep apnea: the most common secondary cause of hypertension associated with resistant hypertension. Hypertension 2011;58:811–7.
51. Marin JM, Agusti A, Villar I, et al. Association between treated and untreated obstructive sleep apnea and risk of hypertension. JAMA 2012;307:2169–76.
52. Barbé F, Durán-Cantolla J, Sánchez-de-la-Torre M, et al, Spanish Sleep And Breathing Network. Effect of continuous positive airway pressure on the incidence of hypertension and cardiovascular events in nonsleepy patients with obstructive sleep apnea: a randomized controlled trial. JAMA 2012;307: 2161–8.
53. Montesi SB, Edwards BA, Malhotra A, et al. The effect of continuous positive airway pressure treatment on blood pressure: a systematic review and meta-analysis of randomized controlled trials. J Clin Sleep Med 2012;8:587–96.
54. Weber SL. Cushing's syndrome attributable to topical use of lotrisone. Endocr Pract 1997;3:14.
55. Nutting CM, Page SR. Iatrogenic Cushing's syndrome due to nasal betamethasone: a problem not to be sniffed at! Postgrad Med J 1995;71:231.
56. Hughes JM, Hichens M, Booze GW, et al. Cushing's syndrome from the therapeutic use of intramuscular dexamethasone acetate. Arch Intern Med 1848; 1986:146.
57. Woods JW. Oral contraceptives and hypertension. Hypertension 1988; 11(3 Pt 2):II11.
58. Chasan-Taber L. Prospective study of oral contraceptives and hypertension among women in the United States. Circulation 1996;94(3):483.

59. Walker MD. Carotid vascular abnormalities in primary hyperparathyroidism. J Clin Endocrinol Metab 2009;94(10):3849.

60. Iglesias P, Acosta M, Sánchez R, et al. Ambulatory blood pressure monitoring in patients with hyperthyroidism before and after control of thyroid function. Clin Endocrinol (Oxf) 2005;63(1):66.

61. Pacak K, Linehan WM, Eisenhofer G, et al. Recent advances in genetics, diagnosis, localization, and treatment of pheochromocytoma. Ann Intern Med 2001; 134:315.

62. Lenders JW, Pacak K, Walther MM, et al. Biochemical diagnosis of pheochromocytoma: which test is best? JAMA 2002;287:1427.

63. Lin JC, Palafox BA, Jackson HA, et al. Cardiac pheochromocytoma: resection after diagnosis by 111-indium octreotide scan. Ann Thorac Surg 1999;67:555.

64. Symplicity HTN-2 Investigators, Esler MD, Krum H, et al. Renal sympathetic denervation in patients with treatment-resistant hypertension (The Symplicity HTN-2 Trial): a randomised controlled trial. Lancet 2010;376(9756):1903.

65. Bisognano JD, Bakris G, Nadim MK, et al. Baroreflex activation therapy lowers blood pressure in patients with resistant hypertension: results from the double-blind, randomized, placebo-controlled Rheos Pivotal Trial. J Am Coll Cardiol 2011;58(7):765.

Renin-Angiotensin-Aldosterone System Inhibition

Overview of the Therapeutic Use of Angiotensin-Converting Enzyme Inhibitors, Angiotensin Receptor Blockers, Mineralocorticoid Receptor Antagonists, and Direct Renin Inhibitors

Kelly Mercier, DO[a], Holly Smith, DO[b], Jason Biederman, DO[b,c],*

KEYWORDS

- Renin • Angiotensin • Aldosterone • Review • Combination • Diabetes
- Kidney disease • Albuminuria

KEY POINTS

- Angiotensin-converting enzyme (ACE) inhibitor or angiotensin receptor blocker (ARB) therapy in hypertensive diabetic patients with macroalbuminuria, microalbuminuria, or normoalbuminuria has been repeatedly shown to improve cardiovascular mortality and reduce the decline in glomerular filtration rate.
- Renin-angiotensin-aldosterone system (RAAS) blockade in normotensive diabetic patients with normoalbuminuria or microalbuminuria cannot be advocated at this time.
- Dual RAAS inhibition with ACE inhibitors plus ARBs or ACE inhibitors plus direct renin inhibitors (DRIs) has failed to improve cardiovascular or renal outcomes but has predisposed patients to serious adverse events.
- An ACE inhibitor or ARB in proteinuric, hypertensive, nondiabetic kidney disease is renoprotective, as long as blood pressure is maintained below 140/90 mm Hg.
- At present, the combination therapy with ACE inhibitors and ARBs or with DRI, aliskiren, and ACE-inhibitor or ARB therapy cannot be advocated for routine use.

Disclosures: None.
[a] Botsford Hospital, 28050 Grand River Avenue, Farmington Hills, MI 48336, USA; [b] Garden City Hospital, 6245 N. Inkster Road, Garden City, MI 48135, USA; [c] Hypertension Nephrology Associates, PC, 18302 Middlebelt Road, Livonia, MI 48152, USA
* Corresponding author. Hypertension Nephrology Associates, PC, 18302 Middlebelt Road, Livonia, Michigan 48152.
E-mail address: jibieder@me.com

CAVEATS

There are 3 points to bear in mind in examining recent literature on inhibition of the renin-angiotensin-aldosterone system (RAAS). First, although the rationale for RAAS inhibition in the therapy for diabetic kidney disease is well established in experimental models of diabetic nephropathy,[1,2] clinically it remains difficult to demonstrate that the effectiveness of these agents is related to a mechanistic effect and is not due to superior blood pressure control. One example is Svensson and colleagues'[3] reanalysis of the HOPE study, demonstrating reduced 24-hour ambulatory blood pressure profiles by ramipril despite the office blood pressures being similar. Hence, the original conclusion that angiotensin-converting enzyme (ACE) inhibition reduced cardiovascular mortality was likely due to better blood pressure control and not to a class effect of ACE inhibitors. Second, nephrology literature commonly relies on the surrogate marker, proteinuria, to predict future outcomes, such as doubling of serum creatinine or development of end-stage renal disease (ESRD). This approach is necessary because of the tremendous time and expense needed to study true renal outcomes, especially as established treatments delay the progression of disease. However, surrogate markers do not always correlate with outcomes. Third, the term diabetic nephropathy currently is reserved for those with renal biopsies showing classic diabetic glomerulosclerosis. Hence, this article uses the more general term diabetic kidney disease, as most clinical trials lack biopsy data.

THERAPEUTIC CONSIDERATIONS WITH ANGIOTENSIN-CONVERTING ENZYME INHIBITOR OR ANGIOTENSIN RECEPTOR BLOCKER COMBINATION MEDICATIONS

ACE inhibitor/thiazide and ARB/thiazide combination medications have been widely used for the treatment of stage 2 hypertension since the Seventh Report of the Joint National Committee on Prevention, Detection, Evaluation, and Treatment of High Blood Pressure.[4] The attractiveness of these combinations was based on recognition that: stage 2 hypertension (blood pressure >160/100 mm Hg) was difficult to treat to goal with monotherapy[5,6]; the side-effect profile is better with 2 antihypertensive medications at lower doses than with the maximal dose of a single medication[7,8]; these combinations are synergistic in their blood pressure–lowering ability[4,7]; and patient adherence is improved by reducing pill burden and the lower cost of thiazide diuretics.[9] These recommendations came on the heels of the ALLHAT study demonstrating the utility of thiazide diuretics in comparison with other classes of antihypertensive therapy.[10] Although these combinations are useful, other factors should be considered before choosing an ACE inhibitor/thiazide or ARB/thiazide combination.

First, the ACCOMPLISH trial demonstrated improved cardiovascular outcomes with benazepril and amlodipine as opposed to benazepril and hydrochlorothiazide.[11] Over the 2.9-year study, faster progression of chronic kidney disease, hypokalemia, and hypotensive episodes was more likely in the benazepril and hydrochlorothiazide arm. Second, hydrochlorothiazide will increase the incidence of impaired glucose tolerance and new-onset diabetes, important considerations in those with or at risk of diabetes mellitus. Lastly, thiazide diuretics also raise total cholesterol and low-density lipoprotein levels, which may be important, especially in younger patients.[12] Despite these potential deleterious effects of thiazides, it must be acknowledged that diuretic use is important, if not imperative, in certain patient populations, such as blacks, and persons with salt-sensitive hypertension, congestive heart failure, or resistant hypertension. Although ACE inhibitor/amlodipine and ARB/amlodipine fixed-dose combinations are more widely used because of their availability, an ACE inhibitor and nondihydropyridine calcium-channel blocker (NDCCB) combination may be preferable, because of the negative chronotropic effects of NDCCBs and their equivalence to β-blockers in primary prevention of cardiovascular events in those without heart failure.[13] In addition, an ACE inhibitor/verapamil combination can reduce proteinuria even further in patients with type 2 diabetes.[14]

DO ANGIOTENSIN RECEPTOR BLOCKERS INCREASE THE RISK OF CANCER?

In 2010, a meta-analysis of 9 trials suggested an association between ARB therapy and cancer risk, primarily lung cancer, over an average follow-up of 4 years.[15] One important pitfall of this study was the lack of access to individual patient data, preventing time-to-event analysis. Subsequently using the Danish national registries with individual patient data, Pasternak and colleagues[16] compared 107,466 new ARB users and 209,692 new ACE-inhibitor users. No increased rate of cancer was found in ARB users, nor was there any increased cancer risk with ongoing ARB exposure among 15 different cancer subgroups, with the exception of male genital cancers. Of importance, no increased risk of lung cancer was observed. The US Food and Drug Administration completed its own analysis in September 2011. Thirty-one trials including 84,461 patients randomized to ARB and 71,355 patients randomized to non-ARB comparators disclosed no increased risk of cancer or cancer-related death over an average follow-up of 39 months.[17]

INHIBITION OF THE RENIN-ANGIOTENSIN-ALDOSTERONE SYSTEM IN HYPERTENSIVE DIABETICS WITH MACROALBUMINURIA

The Collaborative Study Group showed attenuation of proteinuria (>500 mg/24 h) and preservation of glomerular filtration rate (GFR) using the ACE inhibitor, captopril, to treat type 1 diabetic kidney disease in 1993.[18] Several years later, the RENAAL and IDNT studies demonstrated the effectiveness of the ARBs losartan and irbesartan in reducing macroalbuminuria and delaying progression of type 2 diabetic nephropathy.[19,20] Pohl and colleagues[21] later conducted a post hoc analysis of the IDNT, showing a direct correlation between the degree of blood pressure lowering and renal outcomes as long as the systolic blood pressure was maintained higher than 120 mm Hg. Below this threshold, renoprotection was no longer conferred and all-cause mortality rose. Regarding diastolic blood pressure, the HOT trial established a 51% reduction in cardiovascular events when diastolic blood pressure was less than 80 mm Hg in diabetics (**Table 1**).[22]

INHIBITION OF THE RENIN-ANGIOTENSIN-ALDOSTERONE SYSTEM IN HYPERTENSIVE DIABETES WITH MICROALBUMINURIA

Parving and colleagues[23] demonstrated that irbesartan could prevent progression of microalbuminuria to macroalbuminuria in hypertensive type 2 diabetics. Similarly, the MARVAL study compared valsartan with amlodipine in reduction of urinary albumin excretion in type 2 diabetics with urine albumin excretion rates (UAER) of 20 to 200 μg/min and blood pressure less than 180/105 mm Hg. After 24 weeks of treatment, the patients in the valsartan group had significantly less UAER compared with the amlodipine group despite identical reduction in blood pressure.[24] Additional studies have established the role of ACE inhibitors or ARBs in decreasing microvascular and macrovascular events in the treatment of hypertensive diabetic patients.[25,26]

Table 1
Summary of major trials in diabetic kidney disease

Degree of Proteinuria	Trial (year)[Ref.]	Diabetes Type	RAAS Agent	Key Finding
Normoalbuminuria (<30 mg/d or ACR <30 mg/g)				
+ Normotensive	EUCLID (1997)[29]	IDDM	ACE	Did not prevent microalbuminuria
	DIRECT (2009)[30]	Types 1 and 2	ARB	Did not prevent microalbuminuria
	RASS (2009)[31]	Type 1	ACE or ARB	Did not prevent microalbuminuria or diabetic glomerulosclerosis
	ACCORD (2010)[34]	Type 2		SBP <120 did not decrease CV or all-cause mortality and caused greater GFR decline
+ Hypertensive	BENEDICT (2004)[27]	Type 2	ACE	Prevented microalbuminuria
	MICRO-HOPE (2000)[28]	Type 2	ACE	Prevented overt nephropathy,[a] improved CV and total mortality
Microalbuminuria (30–300 mg/d or ACR 30–300 mg/g)				
+ Normotensive	EUCLID (1997)[29]	IDDM	ACE	Improved microalbuminuria
	ACCORD (2010)[34]	Type 2		SBP <120 did not decrease CV or all-cause mortality and caused greater GFR decline
+ Hypertensive	IRMA2 (2001)[23]	Type 2	ARB	Attenuated proteinuria
	MARVAL (2002)[24]	Type 2	ARB	Attenuated proteinuria
Macroalbuminuria (>300 mg/d or ACR >300 mg/g) or UPC >0.5				
+ Hypertensive	Collaborative Study Group (1993)[18]	Type 1	ACE	Prevented ESRD, need for renal transplant, or death
	RENAAL (2001)[19]	Type 2	ARB	Prevented ESRD and doubling of Scr
	IDNT (2001)[20]	Type 2	ARB	Prevented ESRD and doubling of Scr

Abbreviations: ACE, angiotensin-converting enzyme inhibitor; ACR, albumin to creatinine ratio; ARB, angiotensin receptor blocker; CV, cardiovascular; ESRD, end-stage renal disease; GFR, glomerular filtration rate; IDDM, insulin-dependent diabetes mellitus; RAAS, renin-angiotensin-aldosterone system; SBP, systolic blood pressure (mm Hg); Scr, serum creatinine; UPC, urine protein to creatinine ratio.

[a] Overt nephropathy was defined as greater than 300 mg/d of albuminuria, total urine protein excretion greater than 500 mg per 24 hours, or albumin to creatinine ratio greater than 36 mg/mmol and no 24-hour urine result known.

INHIBITION OF THE RENIN-ANGIOTENSIN-ALDOSTERONE SYSTEM IN HYPERTENSIVE DIABETICS WITH NORMOALBUMINURIA

The BENEDICT trial evaluated type 2 diabetics with hypertension and normoalbuminuria to assess prevention of microalbuminuria by using ACE inhibitors versus NDCCB versus both. Treatment with ACE inhibitors, either alone or in combination with NDCCB, delayed the onset of microalbuminuria.[27] The MICRO-HOPE substudy also showed beneficial effects of treatment with RAAS blockade in 3577 diabetic patients, of whom 68% had normoalbuminuria. Patients taking ramipril had fewer adverse events, and 25% had a decreased risk of a primary cardiovascular event after 2 years. In addition, the risk of overt nephropathy and dialysis were decreased with ramipril therapy.[28]

- In summary, ACE-inhibitor or ARB therapy in hypertensive diabetic patients with macroalbuminuria, microalbuminuria, or normoalbuminuria has been repeatedly shown to improve cardiovascular mortality and reduce GFR decline.

INHIBITION OF THE RENIN-ANGIOTENSIN-ALDOSTERONE SYSTEM IN NORMOTENSIVE DIABETICS WITH NORMOALBUMINURIA OR MICROALBUMINURIA

The EUCLID study group followed 500 insulin-dependent diabetics for 2 years to determine whether lisinopril limited progression of renal disease in patients with normoalbuminuria or microalbuminuria. Normotension was defined as systolic blood pressure less than 155 mm Hg and diastolic blood pressure 75 to 90 mm Hg. Overall, microalbuminuric patients benefited from therapy while normoalbuminuric patients did not. However, there were variable results with respect to the intention-to-treat population versus the patients completing the trial.[29] This study, and others like it, were criticized for being underpowered and lacking long-term follow-up. Of note, although lisinopril decreased microalbuminuria on subgroup analysis, the investigators did not measure GFR decline. The DIRECT-Renal analysis was a large, multicenter, international study of more than 5000 patients, all of whom had diabetes and normoalbuminuria. Two of the 3 arms of the study included patients with no history of hypertension, defined as blood pressure less than or equal to 130/85 mm Hg. The third arm involved established hypertensive patients who were well controlled, with blood pressure less than or equal to 160/90 mm Hg. Treatment with candesartan for an average of 5 years failed to prevent microalbuminuria.[30] The RASS study, involving 285 patients with renal biopsy data, failed to demonstrate attenuation of diabetic glomerulosclerosis by ACE inhibitors or ARBs in normotensive, normoalbuminuric type 1 diabetics.[31] To complicate matters, spontaneous regression of microalbuminuria can occur, as shown in a reanalysis of the DCCT/EDIC.[32] The ACCORD study showed improvement in microalbuminuria with intensive blood pressure control (systolic <120 mm Hg). However, there was no change in cardiovascular or all-cause mortality; and intensive blood pressure lowering caused more hypotension, syncope, hyperkalemia, and loss of renal function.[33] The lack of proven benefit in these studies, coupled with concerns from both the post hoc analysis of the IDNT data and the ACCORD study that systolic blood pressures of less than 120 mm Hg in patients with type 2 diabetes are detrimental, lead the authors to conclude that:

- RAAS blockade in normotensive diabetic patients with normoalbuminuria or microalbuminuria cannot be advocated at present.[21,34]

DUAL INHIBITION OF THE RENIN-ANGIOTENSIN-ALDOSTERONE SYSTEM IN DIABETIC KIDNEY DISEASE

Several studies have established the role of ACE inhibitors or ARBs in attenuating albuminuria and decreasing the risk of both ESRD and cardiovascular death. Small studies have demonstrated that dual RAAS blockade can reduce proteinuria and blood pressure further, but have lacked outcome data.[35] The larger ONTARGET trial showed that combining an ACE inhibitors and ARB does not decrease the incidence of cardiovascular events nor does it delay the progression to ESRD, despite reducing proteinuria further. However, it does predispose patients to serious adverse effects; mainly hyperkalemia and acute kidney injury. In ONTARGET, there was actually an increased need for dialysis in patients receiving combination therapy.[36] Likewise, the VA-Nephron-D study was prematurely stopped because of the same adverse events of hyperkalemia and acute kidney injury. Over the 2.2-year median follow-up, the addition of lisinopril to losartan in macroalbuminuric type 2 diabetic patients also failed to improve mortality or cardiovascular outcomes.[37]

Similarly, the DRI aliskiren in combination with losartan has been shown to be effective in reducing proteinuria, but the larger outcome-based study ALTITUDE was terminated after 24 months because of an increased risk of stroke, hyperkalemia, and hypotension without any benefit in cardiovascular or renal outcomes.[38,39]

Finally, the mineralocorticoid receptor antagonist (MRA) spironolactone has been used in concert with ACE inhibitors or ARBs, with successful reduction of proteinuria in diabetic kidney disease.[40] Small studies in nondiabetic kidney disease have found small doses to be safe and even to attenuate GFR decline.[41] MRAs may be useful in those with resistant hypertension, especially with concomitant obesity and/or obstructive sleep apnea.[42,43]

- Dual RAAS inhibition with ACE inhibitors plus ARBs or ACE inhibitors plus DRIs has failed to improve cardiovascular or renal outcomes, but has predisposed patients to serious adverse events.
- Dual blockade with ACE inhibitors or ARBs and MRAs has been safe and renoprotective in small studies.

INHIBITION OF THE RENIN-ANGIOTENSIN-ALDOSTERONE SYSTEM IN NONDIABETIC CHRONIC KIDNEY DISEASE

Several studies have established the benefit of ACE inhibition in nondiabetic kidney disease in retarding the progression of disease, although the effect is more pronounced in proteinuric patients.[44] In the AASK study of black hypertensive patients, ramipril therapy led to a 36% slower mean decline in GFR over 3 years in those with mild proteinuria, but stricter blood pressure control (<140/90 mm Hg) was not more renoprotective.[45,46]

In patients with overt proteinuria without diabetes, GFR decline and proteinuria are attenuated by ACE-inhibitor therapy in comparison with other antihypertensive agents, despite similar blood pressure control.[47] The GISEN group demonstrated a 50% reduction in the risk of doubling of serum creatinine or ESRD in those patients with nephrotic-range proteinuria (>3 g/24 h) by ramipril.[48] The ROAD trial uptitrated ACE-inhibitor or ARB doses to reduce proteinuria to less than 500 to 1000 mg/d and not solely for blood pressure reduction. This strategy reduced proteinuria effectively, slowed GFR decline, and reduced the primary end point of doubling of serum creatinine, ESRD, or death despite comparable blood pressure control.[49]

- ACE inhibitors or ARBs in proteinuric, hypertensive, nondiabetic kidney disease are renoprotective, as long as blood pressure is maintained below 140/90 mm Hg. For nephrotic patients, a blood pressure goal of less than 125/75 mm Hg may yield additional benefit, based on the MDRD study.[50]

Studies of combination ACE-inhibitor and ARB therapy in nondiabetic kidney disease are lacking. It is likely appropriate to extrapolate the results of the ONTARGET trial, although this trial predominantly included patients with mild proteinuria.[36] As the combination is effective in reducing proteinuria further, it remains tempting to use it in those with severe nephrotic syndrome, as the high cardiovascular risk associated with proteinuria must also be considered.[51,52] It is hoped that future studies will evaluate patients with more severe proteinuria.

The DRI aliskiren can lower blood pressure to a greater degree than ACE inhibitors and can lower proteinuria in patients with nondiabetic chronic kidney disease to a similar degree.[53] In addition, the combination of aliskiren and ARB reduces proteinuria more than would be expected from lowering of blood pressure alone.[54] These studies have been small, short-duration studies that observed surrogate markers such as blood pressure and proteinuria. Unfortunately, renal outcome studies will not be forthcoming soon, as results of the ALTITUDE trial in patients with type 2 diabetes found increased cardiovascular risks on combining aliskiren with either ACE inhibitors or ARBs.[39]

- At present, the combination therapy with an ACE inhibitor and an ARB, or with the DRI aliskiren and an ACE inhibitor or ARB, cannot be advocated for routine use.

Another approach to dual RAAS blockade is adding an MRA to either an ACE inhibitor or an ARB. These combinations reduce proteinuria and improve blood pressure, but must be tempered with the increased risk of hyperkalemia, especially in those with advanced chronic kidney disease.[55,56]

INHIBITION OF THE RENIN-ANGIOTENSIN-ALDOSTERONE SYSTEM IN CARDIAC DISEASE AFTER MYOCARDIAL INFARCTION

The current standard of care in postmyocardial infarction (PMI) patients includes RAAS inhibition with either ACE inhibitors or ARBs. Multiple trials demonstrate improvement in left ventricular mass and left ventricular ejection fraction in patients receiving high-dose RAAS inhibition compared with placebo or lower doses of the same medications.[57] In addition to these surrogate markers, ACE-inhibitor therapy PMI reduces mortality in those with heart failure or left ventricular systolic dysfunction, slows progression to severe heart failure in those with left ventricular systolic dysfunction, and reduces the incidence of heart failure.[58,59] Subsequent trials have shown equivalent efficacy of ARBs using these same clinical end points.[60–63]

Trials with PMI patients and high-risk vascular patients show that the combination of ACE inhibitors and ARBs increases the rate of adverse events including symptomatic hypotension, hyperkalemia, discontinuation of medication, and worsening renal failure, without improving survival.[36,63]

Dual RAAS blockade has also been studied in PMI patients with systolic dysfunction by adding the DRI aliskiren to ACE inhibitors or ARBs. Unfortunately, in the ASPIRE study, adding aliskiren to standard PMI therapy, including ACE inhibitors or ARBs, did not further attenuate left ventricular remodeling and was associated with an increase in adverse events.[64]

INHIBITION OF THE RENIN-ANGIOTENSIN-ALDOSTERONE SYSTEM IN CHRONIC HEART FAILURE

RAAS blockade is advantageous in patients with systolic dysfunction. ACE inhibition reduces mortality and hospitalization for heart failure in patients with New York Heart Association (NYHA) class II and III, and decrease mortality in patients with NYHA class IV heart failure.[65,66] In addition, ACE inhibitors reduce the incidence of heart failure in patients with asymptomatic left ventricular dysfunction.[67] ARB therapy in chronic heart failure produces similar benefits, with both reduced mortality and hospitalizations for heart failure in patients with NYHA classes II to IV and left ventricular ejection fraction of less than 40%.[68–70]

ACE-inhibitor and ARB combination therapy does reduce hospitalization for heart failure and cardiovascular death,[70,71] but an increased risk of adverse events including drug discontinuation, hypotension, hyperkalemia, and decline in renal function were also observed.[72] Similarly, in the ASTRONAUT trial, the addition of aliskiren to standard heart-failure therapy did not decrease cardiovascular death or hospitalizations for heart failure, but increased the rate of hyperkalemia, hypotension, and renal impairment.[73]

- RAAS blockade with an ACE inhibitor or an ARB, but not in combination, improves cardiovascular morbidity PMI and in patients with systolic dysfunction.

Contrastingly, MRAs reduce mortality in severe heart failure and reduce cardiovascular death or hospitalization in mild heart failure when combined with either an ACE inhibitor or an ARB.[74–76] As a result, current guidelines recommend aldosterone receptor antagonists in patients with NYHA class II to IV heart failure who have a left ventricular ejection fraction of 35% or less, and also in patients with NYHA class II heart failure who have a history of prior cardiovascular hospitalization. Because of the risk of hyperkalemia and hypotension, the estimated GFR should be greater than 30 mL/min/1.73 m^2 and the potassium level less than 5.0 mEq/L before adding an MRA.[76]

INHIBITION OF THE RENIN-ANGIOTENSIN-ALDOSTERONE SYSTEM IN CEREBROVASCULAR DISEASE

Trials of RAAS inhibition in cardiac disease have found a reduced risk of stroke in patients treated with ACE inhibitors or ARBs. The protective effect of ACE inhibition was further substantiated for prevention of recurrent stroke in the PROGRESS trial.[57,60,77] Subsequently, the ACCOMPLISH trial also found a benefit of ACE inhibitors in reducing cardiovascular events, including nonfatal stroke.[11] ARB studies have been inconclusive in showing a clear benefit in stroke prevention. The TRANSCEND and PRoFESS trials failed to reduce the incidence of subsequent stroke or major cardiovascular events, despite a small reduction in blood pressure in patients treated with ARBs,[78,79] whereas in the MOSES study patients had significantly reduced risk of fatal and nonfatal cerebrovascular accident despite similar blood pressure control.[80]

The ACCESS study evaluated candesartan in the acute phase following the onset of stroke. ARB therapy decreased mortality and vascular events.[81] However, the Scandinavian Candesartan Acute Stroke Trial did not corroborate these findings, as candesartan failed to prevent vascular death, nonfatal stroke, or nonfatal myocardial infarction, or improve functional status when compared with placebo.[82] At present, the data are insufficient to recommend RAAS blockade in the acute stroke period.

REFERENCES

1. Anderson S, Vora JP. Current concepts of renal hemodynamics in diabetes. J Diabet Complications 1995;9(4):304–7.
2. Sochett EB, Cherney DZ, Curtis JR, et al. Impact of renin angiotensin system modulation on the hyperfiltration state in type 1 diabetes. J Am Soc Nephrol 2006;17:1703–9.
3. Svensson P, de Faire U, Sleight P, et al. Comparative effects of ramipril on ambulatory and office blood pressures: a HOPE Substudy. Hypertension 2001;38:e28–32.
4. Chovanian AV, Bakris GL, Black HR, et al. Seventh report of the Joint National Committee on Prevention, Detection, Evaluation, and Treatment of High Blood Pressure. Hypertension 2003;42(6):1206–52.
5. Materson BJ, Reda DJ, Cushman WC, et al. Single-drug therapy for hypertension in men. A comparison of six antihypertensive agents with placebo. The Department of Veterans Affairs Cooperative Study Group on Antihypertensive Agents. N Engl J Med 1993;328(13):914–21.
6. Bakris GL. Maximizing cardiorenal benefit in the management of hypertension: achieve blood pressure goals. J Clin Hypertens 1999;1:141–7.
7. Law MR, Wald NJ, Morris JK, et al. Value of low dose combination treatment with blood pressure lowering drugs: analysis of 354 randomised trials. BMJ 2003; 326(7404):1427.
8. Sica DA. Rationale for fixed-dose combinations in the treatment of hypertension: the cycle repeats. Drugs 2002;62(3):443–62.
9. Greenberg RN. Overview of patient compliance with medication dosing: a literature review. Clin Ther 1984;6:592–9.
10. ALLHAT Officers and Coordinators for the ALLHAT Collaborative Research Group, The Antihypertensive and Lipid-Lowering Treatment to Prevent Heart Attack Trial. Major outcomes in high-risk hypertensive patients randomized to angiotensin-converting enzyme inhibitor or calcium channel blocker vs diuretic: the Antihypertensive and Lipid-Lowering Treatment to Prevent Heart Attack Trial (ALLHAT). JAMA 2002;288:2981–97.
11. Jamerson K, Weber MA, Bakris GL, et al, for the ACCOMPLISH Trial Investigators. Benazepril plus amlodipine or hydrochlorothiazide for hypertension in high-risk patients. N Engl J Med 2008;359(23):2417–28.
12. Grossman E, Verdecchia P, Shamiss A, et al. Diuretic treatment of hypertension. Diabetes Care 2011;34(Suppl 2):S313–9.
13. Black HR, Elliott WJ, Grandits G, et al. Principal results of the Controlled Onset Verapamil Investigation of Cardiovascular End Points (CONVINCE) trial. JAMA 2003;289:2073–82.
14. Rubio-Guerra A, Arceo-Navarro A, Vargas-Ayala G, et al. The effect of trandolapril and its fixed-dose combination with verapamil on proteinuria in normotensive adults with type 2 diabetes. Diabetes Care 2004;27(7):1688–91.
15. Sipahi I, Debanne SM, Rowland DY, et al. Angiotensin-receptor blockade and risk of cancer: meta-analysis of randomised controlled trials. Lancet Oncol 2010;11:627–36.
16. Pasternak B, Svanström H, Callréus T, et al. Use of angiotensin receptor blockers and the risk of cancer. Circulation 2011;123:1729–36.
17. US Food and Drug Administration. FDA drug safety communication: no increase in risk of cancer with certain blood pressure drugs–angiotensin receptor blockers (ARBs). June 2, 2011. Available at: http://www.fda.gov/Drugs/%20DrugSafety/ucm257516.htm. Accessed on January 7, 2014.

18. Lewis EJ, Hunsicker LG, Bain RP, et al, The Collaborative Study Group. The effect of angiotensin-converting-enzyme inhibition on diabetic nephropathy. N Engl J Med 1993;329:1456–62.
19. Brenner BM, Cooper ME, de Zeeuw D, et al, RENAAL Study Investigators. Effects of losartan on renal and cardiovascular outcomes in patients with type 2 diabetes and nephropathy. N Engl J Med 2001;345:861–9.
20. Lewis EJ, Hunsicker LG, Clarke WR, et al, Collaborative Study Group. Renoprotective effect of the angiotensin-receptor antagonist irbesartan in patients with nephropathy due to type 2 diabetes. N Engl J Med 2001;345:851–60.
21. Pohl MA, Blumenthal S, Cordonnier DJ, et al. Independent and additive impact of blood pressure control and angiotensin II receptor blockade on renal outcomes in the irbesartan diabetic nephropathy trial: clinical implications and limitations. J Am Soc Nephrol 2005;16:3027–37.
22. Hansson L, Zanchetti A, Carruthers SG, et al. Effects of intensive blood- pressure lowering and low-dose aspirin in patients with hypertension: principal results of the Hypertension Optimal Treatment (HOT) randomised trial. HOT Study Group. Lancet 1998;351:1755–62.
23. Parving HH, Lehnert H, Bröchner-Mortensen J, et al, Irbesartan in Patients with Type 2 Diabetes and Microalbuminuria Study Group. The effect of irbesartan on the development of diabetic nephropathy in patients with type 2 diabetes. N Engl J Med 2001;345:870–8.
24. Viberti G, Wheeldon N. Microalbuminuria reduction valsartan in patients with type 2 diabetes mellitus: a blood pressure-independent effect. Circulation 2002;106:672–8.
25. Strippoli GF, Craig M, Schena FP, et al. Role of blood pressure targets and specific antihypertensive agents used to prevent diabetic nephropathy and delay its progression. J Am Soc Nephrol 2006;4(Supp 2):S153–5.
26. Barnett AH, Bain SC, Bouter P, et al, for the Diabetics Exposed to Telmisartan and Enalapril Study Group. Angiotensin-receptor blockade versus converting-enzyme inhibition in type 2 diabetes and nephropathy. N Engl J Med 2004; 351:1952–61.
27. Ruggenenti P, Fassi A, Ilieva AP, et al. Bergamo Nephrologic Diabetes Complications Trial (BENEDICT) Investigators: preventing microalbuminuria in type 2 diabetes. N Engl J Med 2004;351:1941–51.
28. HOPE Study Investigators. Effects of ramipril on cardiovascular and microvascular outcomes in people with diabetes mellitus: results of the HOPE study and MICRO-HOPE substudy. Lancet 2000;355:253–9.
29. The Euclid study group. Randomised placebo-controlled trial of lisinopril in normotensive patients with insulin-dependent diabetes and normoalbuminuria or microalbuminuria. Lancet 1997;349:1787–92.
30. Bilous R, Chaturvedi N, Sjolie AK, et al. Effect of candesartan on microalbuminuria and albumin excretion rate in diabetes. Ann Intern Med 2009; 151:11–20.
31. Mauer M, Zinman B, Gardiner R, et al. Renal and retinal effects of enalapril and losartan in type 1 diabetes. N Engl J Med 2009;361.1:40–51.
32. de Boer IH, Rue TC, Cleary PA, et al, for the Diabetes Control and Complications Trial/Epidemiology of Diabetes Interventions and Complications Study Research Group. Long-term renal outcomes of patients with type 1 diabetes mellitus and microalbuminuria: an analysis of the Diabetes Control and Complications Trial/ Epidemiology of Diabetes Interventions and Complications cohort. Arch Intern Med 2011;171(5):412–20.

33. Ismail-Beigi F, Craven T, Banerji MA, et al, for the ACCORD trial group. Effect of intensive treatment of hyperglycaemia on microvascular outcomes in type 2 diabetes: an analysis of the ACCORD randomised trial. Lancet 2010; 376(9739):419–30.

34. Cushman WC, Evans GW, Byington RP, et al, ACCORD Study Group. Effects of intensive blood-pressure control in type 2 diabetes mellitus. N Engl J Med 2010; 362:1575–85.

35. Mogensen C, Neldam S, Tikkanen I, et al, for the CALM study group. Randomised controlled trial of dual blockade of renin-angiotensin system in patients with hypertension, microalbuminuria, and non-insulin dependent diabetes: the candesartan and lisinopril microalbuminuria (CALM) study. BMJ 2000; 321(7274):1440–4.

36. The ONTARGET Investigators. Renal outcomes with telmisartan, ramipril, or both in patients at high vascular risk (the ONTARGET study): a multicenter, randomized, double-blind, controlled trial. Lancet 2008;372:547–53.

37. Fried LF, Emanuele N, Zhang JH, et al, for the VA NEPHRON-D Investigators. Combined angiotensin inhibition for the treatment of diabetic nephropathy. N Engl J Med 2013;369:1892–903.

38. Parving HH, Persson F, Lewis JB, et al, for the AVOID Study Investigators. Aliskiren combined with losartan in type 2 diabetes and nephropathy. N Engl J Med 2008;358:2433–46.

39. Parving HH, Brenner BM, McMurray JJ, et al, for the ALTITUDE Investigators. Cardiorenal end points in a trial of aliskiren for type 2 diabetes. N Engl J Med 2012;367(23):2204–13.

40. Saklayen MG, Gyebi LK, Tasosa J, et al. Effects of additive therapy with spironolactone on proteinuria in diabetic patients already on ACE inhibitor or ARB therapy: results of a randomized, placebo-controlled, double-blind, crossover trial. J Investig Med 2008;56(4):714–9.

41. Bianchi S, Bigazzi R, Campese VM. Long-term effects of spironolactone on proteinuria and kidney function in patients with chronic kidney disease. Kidney Int 2006;70(12):2116–23.

42. Alvarez-Alvarez B, Abad-Cardiel M, Fernandez-Cruz A, et al. Management of resistant arterial hypertension: role of spironolactone versus double blockade of the renin-angiotensin-aldosterone system. J Hypertens 2010;28(11):2329.

43. Nishizaka MK, Zaman MA, Calhoun DA. Efficacy of low-dose spironolactone in subjects with resistant hypertension. Am J Hypertens 2003;16(11 Pt 1):925.

44. Jafar TH, Schmid CH, Landa M, et al. Angiotensin-converting enzyme inhibitors and progression of nondiabetic renal disease. A meta-analysis of patient-level data. Ann Intern Med 2001;135(2):73–87.

45. Agodoa LY, Appel L, Bakris GL, et al, for African American Study of Kidney Disease and Hypertension (AASK) Study Group. Effect of ramipril versus amlodipine on renal outcomes in hypertensive nephrosclerosis: a randomized controlled trial. JAMA 2001;285(21):2719–28.

46. Wright JT Jr, Bakris G, Greene T, et al, for the African American Study of Kidney Disease and Hypertension Study Group. Effect of blood pressure lowering and antihypertensive drug class on progression of hypertensive kidney disease: results from the AASK trial. JAMA 2002;288(19):2421–31.

47. Ruggenenti P, Perna A, Gherardi G, et al, for the GISEN Group. Renal function and requirement for dialysis in chronic nephropathy patients on long-term ramipril: REIN follow-up trial. Gruppo Italiano di Studi Epidemiologici in Nefrologia (GISEN). Ramipril efficacy in nephropathy. Lancet 1998;352(9136):1252–6.

48. The GISEN Group. Randomised placebo-controlled trial of effect of ramipril on decline in glomerular filtration rate and risk of terminal renal failure in proteinuric, non-diabetic nephropathy. Lancet 1997;349:1857–63.

49. Hou FF, Xie D, Zhang X, et al. Renoprotection of Optimal Antiproteinuric Doses (ROAD) Study: a randomized controlled study of benazepril and losartan in chronic renal insufficiency. J Am Soc Nephrol 2007;18(6):1889–98.

50. Klahr S, Levey AS, Beck GJ, et al, Modification of Diet in Renal Disease Study Group. The effects of dietary protein restriction and blood-pressure control on the progression of chronic renal disease. N Engl J Med 1994; 330(13):877–84.

51. Arnlov J, Evans JC, Meigs JB, et al. Low-grade albuminuria and incidence of cardiovascular disease events in nonhypertensive and nondiabetic individuals: the Framingham Heart Study. Circulation 2005;112:969–75.

52. Valmadrid CT, Klein R, Moss SE, et al. The risk of cardiovascular disease mortality associated with microalbuminuria and gross proteinuria in persons with older-onset diabetes mellitus. Arch Intern Med 2000;160(8):1093–100.

53. Lizakowski S, Tylicki L, Renke M, et al. Effect of aliskiren on proteinuria in non-diabetic chronic kidney disease: a double-blind, crossover, randomised, controlled trial. Int Urol Nephrol 2012;44(6):1763–70.

54. Moriyama T, Tsuruta Y, Kojima C, et al. Beneficial effect of aliskiren combined with olmesartan in reducing urinary protein excretion in patients with chronic kidney disease. Int Urol Nephrol 2012;44:841–5.

55. Epstein M. Aldosterone blockade: an emerging strategy for abrogating progressive renal disease. Am J Med 2006;119:912–9.

56. Chrysostomou A, Pedagogos E, MacGregor L, et al. Double-blind, placebo-controlled study on the effect of the aldosterone receptor antagonist spironolactone in patients who have persistent proteinuria and are on long-term angiotensin-converting enzyme inhibitor therapy, with or without an angiotensin II receptor blocker. Clin J Am Soc Nephrol 2006;1(2):256–62.

57. Lonn E, Shaikholeslami R, Yi Q, et al. Effects of ramipril on left ventricular mass and function in cardiovascular patients with controlled blood pressure and with preserved left ventricular ejection fraction: a substudy of the Heart Outcomes Prevention Evaluation (HOPE) trial. J Am Coll Cardiol 2004;43(12):2200–6.

58. Acute Infarction Ramipril Efficacy (AIRE) Study Investigators. Effect of ramipril on mortality and morbidity of survivors of acute myocardial infarction with clinical evidence of heart failure. Lancet 1993;342(8875):821–8.

59. Køber L, Torp-Pedersen C, Carlsen JE, et al. A clinical trial of the angiotensin-converting-enzyme inhibitor trandolapril in patients with left ventricular dysfunction after myocardial infarction. Trandolapril Cardiac Evaluation (TRACE) Study Group. N Engl J Med 1995;333(25):1670–6.

60. Dahlöf B, Devereux RB, Kjeldsen SE, et al, LIFE Study Group. Cardiovascular morbidity and mortality in the Losartan Intervention For Endpoint reduction in hypertension study (LIFE): a randomised trial against atenolol. Lancet 2002; 359(9311):995–1003.

61. Young JB, Dunlap ME, Pfeffer MA, et al. Mortality and morbidity reduction with Candesartan in patients with chronic heart failure and left ventricular systolic dysfunction: results of the CHARM low-left ventricular ejection fraction trials. Circulation 2004;110(17):2618–26.

62. Dickstein K, Kjekshus J, OPTIMAAL Steering Committee of the OPTIMAAL Study Group. Effects of losartan and captopril on mortality and morbidity in high-risk patients after acute myocardial infarction: the OPTIMAAL randomised

trial. Optimal Trial in Myocardial Infarction with Angiotensin II Antagonist Losartan. Lancet 2002;360:752–60.

63. McMurray J, Solomon S, Pieper K, et al. The effect of valsartan, captopril, or both on atherosclerotic events after acute myocardial infarction: an analysis of the Valsartan in Acute Myocardial Infarction Trial (VALIANT). J Am Coll Cardiol 2006;47(4):726–33.

64. Solomon SD, Shin SH, Shah A, et al. Effect of the direct renin inhibitor aliskiren on left ventricular remodeling following myocardial infarction with systolic dysfunction. Eur Heart J 2011;32:1227–34.

65. The SOLVD Investigators. Effect of enalapril on survival in patients with reduced left ventricular ejection fractions and congestive heart failure. N Engl J Med 1991;325(5):293–302.

66. CONSENSUS Trial Study Group. Effects of enalapril on mortality in severe congestive heart failure. Results of the Cooperative North Scandinavian Enalapril Survival Study (CONSENSUS). N Engl J Med 1987;316(23):1429–35.

67. Konstam MA, Kronenberg MW, Rousseau MF, et al. Effects of the angiotensin converting enzyme inhibitor enalapril on the long-term progression of left ventricular dilatation in patients with asymptomatic systolic dysfunction. SOLVD (Studies of Left Ventricular Dysfunction) Investigators. Circulation 1993;88(5 Pt 1):2277–83.

68. Pitt B, Poole-Wilson PA, Segal R, et al. Effect of losartan compared with captopril on mortality in patients with symptomatic heart failure: randomised trial—the Losartan Heart Failure Survival Study ELITE II. Lancet 2000;355:1582–7.

69. Granger CB, McMurray JJ, Yusuf S, et al. Effects of candesartan in patients with chronic heart failure and reduced left-ventricular systolic function intolerant to angiotensin-converting-enzyme inhibitors: the CHARM-Alternative trial. Lancet 2003;362:772–6.

70. McMurray JJ, Ostergren J, Swedberg K, et al. Effects of candesartan in patients with chronic heart failure and reduced left-ventricular systolic function taking angiotensin-converting-enzyme inhibitors: the CHARM-Added trial. Lancet 2003;362:767–71.

71. Carson P, Tognoni G, Cohn JN. Effect of Valsartan on hospitalization: results from Val-HeFT. J Card Fail 2003;9(3):164–71.

72. Phillips CO, Kashani A, Ko DK, et al. Adverse effects of combination angiotensin II receptor blockers plus angiotensin-converting enzyme inhibitors for left ventricular dysfunction. Arch Intern Med 2007;167:1930–6.

73. Gheorghiade M, Böhm M, Greene SJ, et al, ASTRONAUT Investigators and Coordinators. Effect of aliskiren on postdischarge mortality and heart failure readmissions among patients hospitalized for heart failure: the ASTRONAUT randomized trial. JAMA 2013;309(11):1125–35.

74. Zannad F, McMurray JJ, Krum H, et al, EMPHASIS-HF Study Group. Eplerenone in patients with systolic heart failure and mild symptoms. N Engl J Med 2011;364(1):11–21.

75. Pitt B, Zannad F, Remme WJ, et al. The effect of spironolactone on morbidity and mortality in patients with severe heart failure. Randomized Aldactone Evaluation Study Investigators. N Engl J Med 1999;341(10):709–17.

76. Yancy CW, Jessup M, Bozkurt B, et al. 2013 ACCF/AHA guideline for the management of heart failure: a report of the American College of Cardiology Foundation/American Heart Association Task Force on Practice Guidelines. Circulation 2013;128(16):e240–327. Available at: http://circ.ahajournals.org/content/early/2013/06/03/CIR.0b013e31829e8807.citation.

77. PROGRESS Collaborative Group. Randomised trial of a perindopril-based blood-pressure-lowering regimen among 6,105 individuals with previous stroke or transient ischaemic attack. Lancet 2001;358(9287):1033–41.

78. The Telmisartan Randomised AssessmeNt Study in ACE iNtolerant subjects with cardiovascular Disease (TRANSCEND) Investigators. Effects of the angiotensin-receptor blocker telmisartan on cardiovascular events in high-risk patients intolerant to angiotensin-converting enzyme inhibitors: a randomised controlled trial. Lancet 2008;372(9644):1174–83.

79. Yusuf S, Phil D, Diener HC, et al, for the PRoFESS study group. Telmisartan to prevent recurrent stroke and cardiovascular events. N Engl J Med 2008;359: 1225–37.

80. Schrader J, Lüders S, Kulschewski A, et al. Morbidity and mortality after stroke, eprosartan compared with nitrendipine for secondary prevention: principal results of a prospective randomized controlled study (MOSES). Stroke 2005; 36(6):1218–26.

81. Schrader J, Lüders S, Kulschewski A, et al, Acute Candesartan Cilexetil Therapy in Stroke Survivors Study Group. The ACCESS Study: evaluation of Acute Candesartan Cilexetil Therapy in Stroke Survivors. Stroke 2003;34(7):1699–703.

82. Hornslien AG, Sandset EC, Bath PM, et al, Scandinavian Candesartan Acute Stroke Trial Study Group. Effects of candesartan in acute stroke on cognitive function and quality of life: results from the Scandinavian Candesartan Acute Stroke Trial. Stroke 2013;44(7):2022–4.

Evaluation of Acute Kidney Injury in the Hospital Setting

Parham Eftekhari, DO, MSc

KEYWORDS

- Acute kidney injury • Hospital-acquired acute kidney injury
- Hospital-acquired acute renal failure • Renal failure • Nosocomial acute kidney injury
- Nosocomial renal failure

KEY POINTS

- Incidence of hospital-acquired acute kidney injury (AKI) has been recently estimated at 22% and is most prevalent in the intensive care unit.
- Assessment of renal function in the hospital setting should entail evaluation of serum creatinine, estimation of glomerular filtration rate (GFR), and urine output.
- Distinguishing among the 3 categories of AKI (pre-renal, acute tubular necrosis [ATN], post-renal) will help to differentiate potential causative factors and guide a more effective management plan.
- In the hospital setting, the most common cause of AKI is ATN, commonly caused by prolonged hypotension, sepsis, nephrotoxic medications, and contrast nephropathy.
- Important patient risk factors for development of AKI in the hospital setting include age greater than 65, sepsis, chronic kidney disease, diabetes mellitus, HIV, and surgery.
- General principles of AKI management include optimizing hemodynamic status, adjusting drug dosages for appropriate GFR, recognizing potential nephrotoxic medications, and treating acute electrolyte disorders.

NATURE OF THE PROBLEM

Acute renal failure now increasingly referred to as acute kidney injury (AKI), is a syndrome characterized by decreased glomerular filtration with a wide spectrum of severity.[1–3] AKI is generally defined by the abrupt loss of kidney function, resulting in the retention of urea and other nitrogenous waste products. Other common clinical and laboratory manifestations of AKI include decreased urine output, metabolic acidosis, and increased potassium and phosphate concentrations.[1–3]

Globally, the incidence of AKI in the hospital setting continues to rise and is associated with significant mortality. The incidence of AKI in the hospital setting has been

Broward Health Medical Center, Nova Southeastern University College of Osteopathic Medicine, 6301 Southwest 112 Street, Miami, FL 33156, USA
E-mail address: Peftekh@gmail.com

Prim Care Clin Office Pract 41 (2014) 779–802
http://dx.doi.org/10.1016/j.pop.2014.08.005
0095-4543/14/$ – see front matter © 2014 Elsevier Inc. All rights reserved.

noted to be as high as 22% with up to 67% occurring in intensive care units (ICU).[4–9] More importantly, the development of AKI is independently associated with high mortality rates, increased length of stay, and risk of developing permanent chronic kidney disease (CKD).[4–7,9–11]

DEFINITION OF ACUTE KIDNEY INJURY

More than 30 definitions of AKI have been acknowledged in the medical literature. In 2002, the Acute Dialysis Quality Initiative expert panel created a uniform, universal definition of AKI known as the RIFLE criteria for the diagnosis, treatment, and prevention of AKI.[3] RIFLE is an acronym that standardizes a definition for the different spectrums of renal impairment according to risk, injury, failure, loss, and end-stage kidney disease (**Fig. 1**). The principle aim of this criterion is to heighten awareness for the diagnosis of early acute renal injury with goal of promoting therapeutic interventions to avoid progression of AKI.[12] Furthermore, hospitalized patients who are categorized in a higher RIFLE class tend to have higher mortality rates, especially in the ICU.[4,8,12,13]

ASSESSMENT OF KIDNEY FUNCTION IN THE HOSPITAL SETTING

Before addressing causality, diagnosis, and therapeutic modalities for AKI, clinicians should first appreciate how to properly assess renal function in the hospital setting. For example, drug administration, including antibiotics and other therapeutic treatments, often require dose adjustments according to patients' estimated renal function.[14,15]

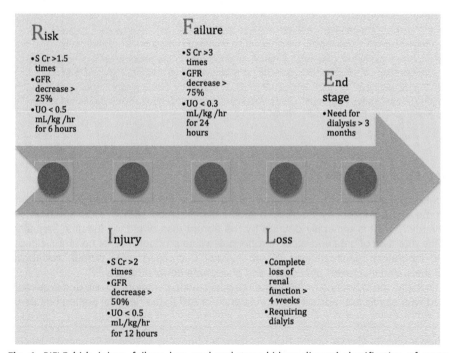

Fig. 1. RIFLE (risk, injury, failure, loss, and end-stage kidney disease) classification of acute renal failure. GFR, glomerular filtration rate; S Cr, serum creatinine; UO, urine output. (*Data from* Bellomo R, Kellum JA, Ronco C, et al. Acute renal failure – definition, outcome measures, animal models, fluid therapy, and information technology needs: the second international consensus of the Acute Dialysis Quality Initiative (ADQI) group. Crit Care 2004;8:R204–12.)

In the hospital setting, serum creatinine is an important and convenient laboratory marker that can help to identify patients suffering from acute or chronic renal disease. However, measurement of serum creatinine alone is not the most accurate way of evaluating a patient's true renal function, because numerous factors influence the baseline level of serum creatinine production, including age, sex, dietary intake, and muscle mass.[16–18] Therefore, for the same degree of renal failure, serum creatinine measurements will tend to be lower in specific patient populations, such as the elderly, malnourished patients with terminal conditions, and those with cirrhosis. In the ICU setting, patients will also tend to have decreased creatinine production because of prolonged immobilization, malnutrition, decreased muscle mass, or hemodilution from intravenous (IV) fluid administration.[8,16,19,20] Hence, a frail elderly woman with a slightly elevated serum creatinine will actually have an impaired renal function, which is probably much worse compared with a younger male with similar laboratory results. As such, evaluation of renal function by serum creatinine alone may lead care providers to misinterpret a patient's true degree of renal function with subsequent risk of developing nosocomial AKI.[18,21]

The glomerular filtration rate (GFR) serves as better tool for evaluating renal function. However, the GFR cannot be measured directly and it is often determined through the use of rapid estimation equations that are readily available online or through the use of mobile devices. The normal GFR is approximately 130 mL/min/1.73 m^2 in younger men and 120 mL/min/1.73 m^2 in younger women.[21] Three common GFR calculators used in hospital setting, include the Cockcroft-Gault equation, Modification of Diet in Renal Disease, and the Chronic Kidney Disease-Epidemiology Equation. These equations take into account important patient variable including age, sex, and serum creatinine level in determining a patient's estimated GFR.[14,18,21] Therefore, health care providers should evaluate changes in both the serum creatinine and corresponding GFR measurements when evaluating a patient's renal function in the hospital setting, especially with regard to medication dose adjustments.[14,15,21]

CATEGORIES OF ACUTE KIDNEY INJURY

Early recognition and management of AKI is crucial in the hospital setting. Once identified, differentiating the subtype of AKI among 3 different categories will help to determine more effective diagnostic and treatment modalities. The etiology of AKI has traditionally been divided into 3 broad categories based on the anatomic location of the injury (Fig. 2). The most common cause of AKI in the hospital setting is acute tubular necrosis (ATN), followed by pre-renal causes.[22,23]

Medication-Induced Acute Kidney Injury

One of the most common and important causes of iatrogenic AKI in the hospital setting is medication adverse effects. This occurs through many different mechanisms involving all 3 categories of AKI including reduction in renal perfusion (pre-renal), direct cell nephrotoxicity (ATN), adverse allergic reaction (acute interstitial nephritis [AIN]), and medication-induced urinary retention (post-renal).[23–25] A detailed list of medications commonly associated with AKI is also outlined in Table 1.

In general, risk factors that increases patient vulnerability to medication induced AKI in the hospital setting are categorized as (Fig. 3)[29]:

- Patient specific
- Kidney specific
- Drug specific

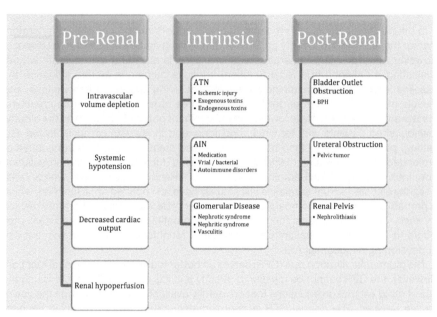

Fig. 2. Categories of acute kidney injury in hospitalized patients. AIN, acute interstitial nephritis; ATN, acute tubular necrosis; BPH, benign prostatic hypertrophy. (*Data from* Nolan C, Anderson R. Hospital acquired acute renal failure. J Am Soc Nephrol 1998;9:710–18; and Thadhani R, Pascual M, Bonventre JV. Acute renal failure. N Engl J Med 1996;344:1448–60.)

Table 1
Common medications responsible for AKI in the hospital setting

Pre-Renal Injury	ATN	Interstitial Nephritis
Renin-angiotensin blockers: ACE-I, ARB	*Antibiotics:* Aminoglycosides, amphotericin B, colistin, vancomycin toxicity	*Antibiotics:* Penicillin, cephalosporin, fluoroquinolones, sulfonamides, rifampin, vancomycin NSAIDs: Ibuprofen, naproxen
NSAIDs: Ibuprofen, naproxen	HIV medication: Tenfovoir, adefovir, cidofovir	*Antiviral:* Acyclovir, gancyclovir
COX-2 inhibitors: Celecoxib	*Iodinated radiocontrast:* CT scan/angiogram, cardiac catheterization	*Gout medication:* Allopurinol
Diuretics: Loop diuretics; thiazide diuretics	*Statins* (lovastatin, etc): Rhabdomyolysis *Colchicine:* Rhabdomyolysis	*Proton pump inhibitors:* Omeprazole, lansoprazole
Immunomodulators: Tacrolimus, cyclosporine	*Bisphosphonates:* Alendronate, zolendronate	Lithium
	Chemotherapy: Cisplatin, carboplatin	Mesalamine
		Anti-epileptic: Valproic acid, phenytoin

Abbreviations: ACE-I, angiotensin converting enzyme inhibitors; AKI, acute kidney injury; ARB, angiotensin receptor blockers; ATN, acute tubular necrosis; COX-2, cyclooxygenase 2 inhibitors; CT, computed tomography; NSAID, nonsteroidal anti-inflammatory drugs.
    Data from Refs.[24,26–28]

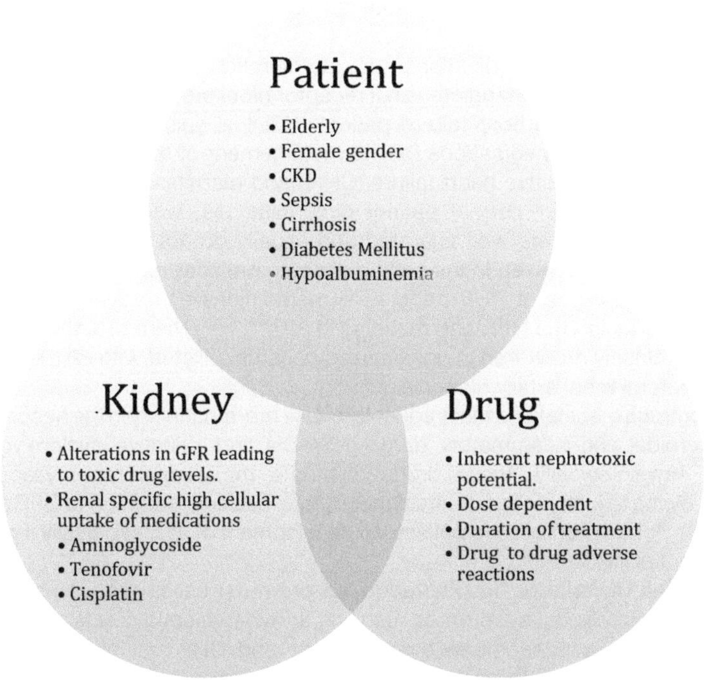

Patient

- Elderly
- Female gender
- CKD
- Sepsis
- Cirrhosis
- Diabetes Mellitus
- Hypoalbuminemia

Kidney

- Alterations in GFR leading to toxic drug levels.
- Renal specific high cellular uptake of medications
- Aminoglycoside
- Tenofovir
- Cisplatin

Drug

- Inherent nephrotoxic potential.
- Dose dependent
- Duration of treatment
- Drug to drug adverse reactions

Fig. 3. Specific risk factors for development of drug-induced acute kidney injury. CKD, chronic kidney disease; GFR, glomerular filtration rate. (*Data from* Schetz M, Dasta J, Goldstein S, et al. Drug-induced acute kidney injury. Curr Opin Crit Care 2005;11:555–65; and Perazella MA. Renal vulnerability to drug toxicity. Clin J Am Soc Nephrol 2009;4:1275–83.)

Important patient risk factors include advanced age and female gender, which are associated with decreased muscle mass and total body water. This can often lead to unrecognized impaired GFR owing to a lower level of measured serum creatinine in the setting of AKI or volume depletion.[24,29] Comorbid conditions that cause significant hypoalbuminemia can also lead to reduced effective circulating blood volume, predisposing such patients to hypovolemic pre-renal injury. Low serum albumin concentrations can lead to reduced drug-binding capability to proteins, which may potentially increase free circulating drug level, thus raising risk of nephrotoxicity.[29]

Some kidney-specific risk factors include alterations in the GFR as well as the degree of cellular uptake and excretion of medications handled by renal tubular cells. For example, aminoglycosides have a unique propensity for higher intracellular proximal tubular entry through specific transport and endocytosis pathways in proximal tubular cells, leading to increased intracellular drug concentration and nephrotoxicity.[24,29]

Two important drug-specific factors include dosing and duration of medication therapy. For example, vancomycin and aminoglycosides are 2 common hospital medications that require close pharmacokinetic monitoring by antibiotic serum trough levels for proper dose adjustments, especially in the setting of AKI.

Pre-renal Acute Kidney Injury

In the hospital setting, pre-renal AKI commonly results from acute renal hypoperfusion, with or without systemic arterial hypotension. This is often a reversible insult as a result of volume depletion from inadequate fluid intake or extrarenal fluid losses such as gastrointestinal bleeding, nausea, vomiting, pancreatitis, and hypoalbuminemia.[30,31]

Commonly prescribed medications such as diuretics and angiotensin-converting enzyme inhibitors (ACE-I) or angiotensin II receptor blockers (ARB) can also contribute to renal hypoperfusion in hospitalized patients. Clinical guidelines recommend pre-scribing ACE-I or ARB medications for the management of medical conditions such as hypertension, congestive heart failure (CHF), and diabetes mellitus (DM)-induced microalbuminuria. Under normal patient circumstances, where renal perfusion is adequate, these drugs are well tolerated and usually do not pose a significant risk for developing AKI. However, in the setting of acute illnesses resulting in hypovolemia or hypotension, the use of ACE-I and ARB medications can adversely affect renal perfusion by reducing the GFR and resulting in AKI.[25,30,31] Therefore, their use should be limited or closely monitored in hospitalized patients afflicted with AKI, especially in cases of bilateral renal artery stenosis.[25,31–33]

Other common medications that frequently cause pre-renal injury in the hospital setting are nonsteroidal anti-inflammatory drugs (NSAIDs) and selective cyclooxygenase-2 inhibitors. Physiologically, these drugs attenuate the normal renal vasodilatation response, owing to inhibition of prostaglandins, thus causing reduction of GFR and renal perfusion.[34–36] This predisposes patients to development of AKI, especially if combined with an ACE-I or ARB.[25,30,31,36]

Although the majority of hospital acquired pre-renal cases are owing to volume depletion, certain clinical syndromes resulting in hypervolemia can lead to pre-renal AKI as well, such as decompensated cirrhosis and CHF.[23,37–39] Decompensated cirrhosis can lead to hepatorenal syndrome, wherein severe portal hypertension trig-gers endogenous arterial vasodilators to cause a maladaptive progressive decline in renal perfusion and severe AKI.[37] Large volume paracentesis without administration of IV albumin can also precipitate AKI.[38]

Acute decomposition of cardiac function, as seen in advanced CHF or cardiogenic shock, can also lead to pre-renal AKI owing to maladaptive neurohormonal responses that cause progressive renal hypoperfusion known as the cardiorenal syndrome. In contrast with volume-depleted pre-renal patients, CHF patients with the cardiorenal syndrome require diuretic therapy to improve cardiac function that will subsequently improve renal perfusion.[39]

Therefore, regardless of the cause, the key to reversing and treating pre-renal AKI is to optimize volume status to achieve a state of euvolemia, while addressing the acute medical conditions. If not corrected in a timely manner, a prolonged pre-renal insult may lead to more serious intrinsic kidney injury, known as ATN.

Intrinsic Acute Kidney Injury

Intrinsic AKI, in contrast with pre-renal, involves structural injury to the renal paren-chyma and can be subdivided into 4 categories according to anatomic site of renal injury: Tubular (ATN), interstitial (AIN), glomerular, and vascular diseases (**Fig. 4**).[28,31,36]

Acute Tubular Necrosis

The majority of intrinsic AKI cases in the hospital setting are secondary to ATN.[22] The most common cause of ATN is prolonged renal cell ischemia as a result of ongoing pre-renal insults. Risk factors for the development of ischemic ATN include a preexist-ing history of CKD, DM, CHF, cirrhosis, and sepsis.[23,26,40]

Exogenous toxins responsible for ATN are most commonly medications such as aminoglycosides, colistin, amphotericin B, or IV iodinated contrast agents (see

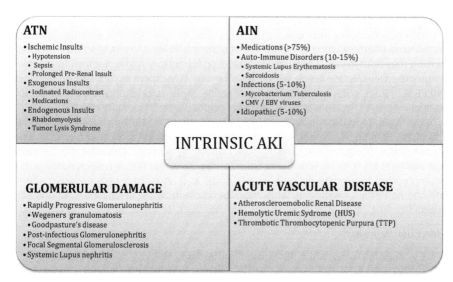

Fig. 4. Important causes of intrinsic acute kidney injury (AKI). ATN, acute tubular necrosis; AIN, acute interstitial nephritis; CMV, cytomegalovirus; EBV, Ebstein-Barr virus. (*Data from* Refs.[28,31,54])

Table 1).[24,26–28] The duration of medication use and dosing periods are also important drug-specific risk factors for ATN.

With increasing use of diagnostic imaging in the hospital, IV iodinated radiocontrast agents are also a common cause of ATN, known as contrast-induced nephropathy (CIN). Computed tomography (CT), angiograms, and cardiac catheterization commonly use iodinated IV contrast agents that are known to cause ATN. The mechanisms for contrast nephropathy include renal vasoconstriction leading to renal ischemia and direct cellular toxicity.[41,42] The ATN seen in CIN appears 24 to 48 hours after injection of contrast media and under optimal circumstances, is usually characterized by improvement in renal function within 1 week.[42] Important risk factors for the development of CIN include a history of CKD, DM, multiple myeloma, volume depletion, and concurrent administration of nephrotoxic medications.[43] Additional risk factors include the total dose of IV contrast administered and use of higher osmolar agents.[41–43] The use of lower osmole contrast (500–850 mosmol/kg) or iso-osmolal (approximately 290 mosmol/kg) agents has been shown to reduce risk of developing CIN.[41–43]

In comparison with iodinated contrast agents, gadolinium used in magnetic resonance imaging is less likely to be associated with AKI. Instead, the use of gadolinium in advanced CKD and dialysis patients has been linked to the development of a unique skin disorder called nephrogenic systemic fibrosis.[44] However, there are emerging data from studies that gadolinium-based contrast media can be associated with nephrotoxicity when given at high doses. Therefore, magnetic resonance imaging gadolinium should also be avoided in patients suffering from severe AKI, advanced CKD with a GFR of less than 30 mL/min, and end-stage renal disease on dialysis.[43–45]

The remaining ATN cases result from endogenously produced nephrotoxic substances, such as myoglobin and uric acid. Two common cases in hospital setting include rhabdomyolysis and tumor lysis syndrome.

Rhabdomyolysis is a potentially life-threatening syndrome resulting from massive breakdown of skeletal muscles causing myoglobin-induced tubular injury and AKI.

Etiologies include crush injury, alcohol abuse, cocaine, and medications such as statins and colchicine. For example, some drugs such as cyclosporine, erythromycin, and fenofibrates interfere with the clearance of statins and lead to elevated plasma levels causing rhabdomyolysis. Diagnosis is based on laboratory findings showing elevated serum creatinine kinase levels with myoglobinuria. Treatment is focused on administration of IV fluid, such as isotonic normal saline, while normalizing electrolyte abnormalities including hyperkalemia, metabolic acidosis, and hypocalcemia.[46,47]

Tumor lysis syndrome is an oncologic emergency caused by massive tumor cell lysis after initiation of chemotherapy, resulting in the precipitation of uric acid in renal tubules and subsequent AKI. This is most commonly seen with treatment of hematologic cancers such as leukemia and lymphomas. To avoid tumor lysis syndrome, it is recommended to hydrate patients with IV fluids and administer hypouricemic agents with chemotherapy treatments while monitoring electrolytes, creatinine, and uric acid levels.[48]

Interstitial Nephritis

AIN is characterized by acute interstitial inflammatory injury by macrophages, B cells, and T cells with an abrupt onset of AKI.[28] The overwhelming majority of cases are owing to antibiotics, including penicillin and cephalosporins, but many other medications have recently been attributed to causing AIN (see **Table 1**).[49,50]

Drug-induced AIN should be suspected with the abrupt onset of nonoliguric AKI after initiation of a new drug, especially in patients admitted without any prior history of renal failure or risk factors for other categories of AKI. The onset of drug-induced AIN is typically seen 2 to 5 days after initiation of the offending drug. Traditionally, patients with drug-induced AIN were reported to have symptoms and/or signs of an allergic-type reaction, including rash, fever, and eosinophilia, but the absence of any of these does not exclude this diagnosis.[49,50] Urine studies can reveal eosinophiluria with white blood cell casts.[49,51] However, the sensitivity of urinary eosinophils for diagnosis of AIN remains relatively low.[51] Eosinophiluria can be also found in a variety of conditions other than AIN, including transplant rejection, pyelonephritis, prostatitis, cystitis, atheroembolic disease, and rapidly progressive glomerulonephritis.[51] If there is a diagnostic dilemma, a kidney biopsy can be done. In such cases, it may be necessary to consult a nephrologist to review the clinical case and to discuss the risk and benefits of this invasive procedure with the patient. Treatment entails abrupt recognition and discontinuation of the offending agent and, in certain cases, initiation of steroid therapy.[52]

Glomerular Disease

Glomerular diseases are less common causes of hospital acquired AKI. However, early diagnosis and intervention can make a significant impact on improving patient outcomes. **Fig. 4** outlines some of the glomerular diseases known to cause abrupt onset of severe AKI in the hospital setting.[53]

Glomerular diseases are generalized into 2 categories—nephrotic and nephritic syndrome (**Fig. 5**).[53,54] Clinicians should be aware of important risk factors that can cause glomerular damage include HIV, systemic lupus erythematosus, DM, and vasculitis. Urine findings suggestive of glomerular damage include proteinuria and hematuria, and dysmorphic red cell casts.[53,54]

In the hospital setting, nephritic syndromes are more often associated with acute proliferative glomerular damage and subsequent AKI. For example, rapidly progressive glomerulonephritis is categorized as a nephritic syndrome causing extensive glomerular damage with a rapid decrease in the GFR over a short period of time.

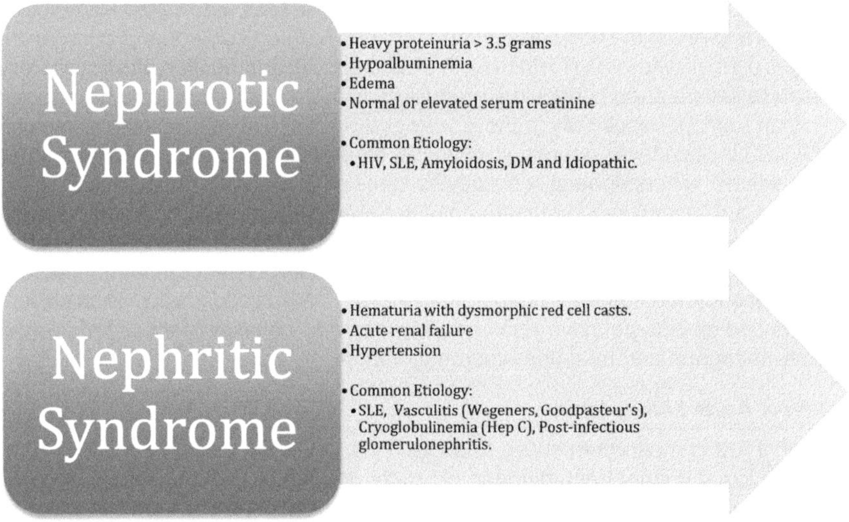

Nephrotic Syndrome
- Heavy proteinuria > 3.5 grams
- Hypoalbuminemia
- Edema
- Normal or elevated serum creatinine
- Common Etiology:
  - HIV, SLE, Amyloidosis, DM and Idiopathic.

Nephritic Syndrome
- Hematuria with dysmorphic red cell casts.
- Acute renal failure
- Hypertension
- Common Etiology:
  - SLE, Vasculitis (Wegeners, Goodpasteur's), Cryoglobulinemia (Hep C), Post-infectious glomerulonephritis.

Fig. 5. Evaluation of glomerular diseases in the hospital setting. DM, diabetes mellitus; Hep C, hepatitis C; SLE, systemic lupus erythematosus. (*Data from* Hricik D, Chung-Park M, Sedor JR. Glomerulonephritis. N Engl J Med 1998;339:888–99; and Floege J, Feehally J. Introduction to glomerular disease: clinical presentations. In: Floege J, Johnson RJ, Feehally J, editors. Comprehensive clinical nephrology. 4th edition. Philadelphia: WB Saunders; 2010. p. 193–207.)

Wegener and Goodpasture syndromes are 2 rapidly progressive glomerulonephritis vasculitis syndromes that present with new onset of hematuria, proteinuria, and severe AKI along with other serious systemic complications, such as pulmonary hemorrhage presenting as hemoptysis. Aggressive treatment with steroids, immune-modulating drugs, and plasma exchange can help to preserve renal function.[54,55]

Infections have also been associated with the development of glomerulonephritis in the hospital setting.[54,56] Bacteremia with streptococcal or staphylococcal infections, especially in cases of endocarditis, can lead to acute postinfectious glomerulonephritis with acute onset of hematuria, proteinuria, and AKI.[56] Lupus (systemic lupus erythematosus) patients with renal disease can have either nephritic or nephrotic syndromes. However, proliferative lupus nephritis commonly presents as nephritic syndrome with acute onset of AKI, hematuria, and variable proteinuria, and may progress to permanent renal failure. Based on renal biopsy, treatment often entails use of immune-modulating drugs, including steroids.[53,54]

Acute Vascular Damage

Renal atheroembolic disease, commonly referred to as cholesterol crystal embolization, is seen in patients with advanced atherosclerotic disease who experience abrupt onset of AKI 1 to 2 weeks after percutaneous cardiac catheterization or vascular surgery. The time of AKI onset is later compared with CIN, which often occurs 1 to 2 days after IV contrast imaging. A common clinical manifestation of atheroembolic disease includes new onset of purple or gangrenous skin discoloration of 1 or more extremities, known as livedo reticularis. Laboratory findings may reveal eosinophilia, eosinophiluria, and hypocomplementemia.[57] Unfortunately, there is no specific treatment beside supportive care.

A rare but important life-threatening microvascular disease associated with multiorgan failure and AKI in the hospital setting is thrombotic thrombocytopenic purpura and hemolytic uremic syndrome (TTP/HUS). Profound platelet aggregation and fibrin formation lead to severe endothelial injury producing arteriolar microthrombi, which causes end-organ damage, especially in the kidney and brain.[58] The classic clinical features of TTP/HUS include fever, neurologic changes, renal failure, and micro-angiopathic hemolytic anemia with peripheral schistocytes in the setting of thrombocytopenia. However, fever and neurologic symptoms may not always be present.[59] Bloody diarrhea is more often seen in HUS cases. More than 40% of TTP/HUS cases are idiopathic, whereas secondary causes include autoimmune disorders (systemic lupus erythematosus), malignancy, infections (HIV), and pregnancy.[58,60] Medications such as calcineurin inhibitors and clopidogrel have also been implicated as causative factors.[60] Failure to promptly recognize and treat this syndrome dramatically increases risk of mortality.

Post-renal Acute Kidney Injury

Post-renal AKI is most often owing to acute urinary outflow obstruction either at the site of the lower urinary tract (bladder, prostate, urethra) or upper urinary tract (renal pelvis and ureters). Common causes of lower tract obstruction include benign prostatic hypertrophy (BPH), prostate cancer, and urinary retention as seen with neurogenic bladder.[2,61,62] In elderly men, BPH remains the most common cause of acute urinary retention. In addition, urinary retention can also occur from neurologic interruption of bladder tone as seen in spinal cord injuries, diabetic neuropathy, and patients with cerebrovascular accidents. Medications commonly implicated in causing urinary retention are listed in **Table 2**.[62]

The clinical presentation of post-renal AKI depends on the site of obstruction, the degree of obstruction, and the rapidity with which obstruction develops. Patients often present with variable changes in urine output, voiding difficulties, or oliguria in severe cases. A distended bladder and flank pain in the setting of AKI are highly suggestive of post-renal AKI. The diagnostic modality of choice is a renal bladder ultrasound. If nephrolithiasis is suspected, noncontrast CT can reveal the anatomic location and severity of disease.[2,61] Early identification and treatment of post-renal AKI is essential because relief of obstructive causes often results in recovery of renal function.

SPECIFIC HOSPITALIZED PATIENTS AT RISK FOR ACUTE KIDNEY INJURY

Prevention of AKI and recognition of early signs are essential in the hospital setting. It is important to recognize specific patients who are at greatest risk for developing AKI. **Fig. 6** outlines specific patient populations that are at high risk for developing AKI.

Geriatric Population

In the United States, geriatric patients age 65 and older represent a large percent of hospitalized adults. Data from the United States Renal Data System in 2013 revealed the rate of AKI in hospital setting to be significantly higher in elderly patients, aged 66 years or greater, compared with all other age groups.[65]

Some of the renal-specific physiologic factors that predispose geriatric patients to AKI include advanced glomerulosclerosis of the kidneys, chronic microvasculature ischemic changes in the cortical glomeruli, and interstitial fibrosis. For example, the advanced interstitial fibrosis seen in the geriatric kidney can lead to maladaptive sodium conservation in renal tubules and loss of urinary concentrating and diluting ability.[66,67] Clinically, such changes result in an increased risk of developing acute volume depletion and hypovolemia, especially in the setting of sepsis, gastrointestinal losses,

Table 2
Clinical evaluation and expected urine examination for AKI in hospital setting

Category of AKI	Clinical History	Urine Findings
Pre-renal	Volume depletion	
	Gastrointestinal losses	FENa <1%
	Diuretic overuse	FEUrea <35%
	Severe burn	
	Concurrent use of ACE-I, ARB, or NSAID.	Urine sodium <20 mmol/L
	Medication induced hypotension	BUN/Cr ratio >20:1
	Malnutrition: Low serum albumin	Urinalysis: High specific gravity, absence of pathologic casts.
	Advanced CHF	Urine sediment bland
	• Cardiorenal syndrome	• Absence of dysmorphic red cell casts.
	Advanced Cirrhosis	
	• Hepatorenal syndrome	• Absence of dark granular casts.
Intrinsic		
ATN	Nephrotoxic medications, sepsis, contrast induced nephropathy, trauma, recent chemotherapy causing TLS.	FENa >2% FEUrea >35% Urine Na>20 mmol/L BUN/Cr ratio 10:1 Urine sediments: Muddy brown casts, myoglobinuria
AIN	Medication use, especially antibiotics	FENa >1% Urine sodium >20 mmol/L Urine sediment: White blood cell casts, eosinophiluria
Glomerular diseases	Proteinuria, hematuria, DM, lupus, HIV, vasculitis, hepatitis C, multiple myeloma, amyloidosis, recent throat infection or endocarditis.	FENa <1% or greater Urine sediment active: Dysmorphic red cells, mixed cell casts
Vascular damage	Thrombocytopenia (TTP/HUS), atherosclerosis with recent PCTA or surgery.	FENa >1% or <1%, hematuria
Post-renal	Oliguria, urinary urgency, gross hematuria, bladder distention, flank pain, history of pelvic or prostate disease, neurologic disease, UTI.	FENa variable; urine sodium often >20 mmol/L; variable hematuria or WBC in urine.

Abbreviations: ACE-I, angiotensin converting enzyme inhibitors; AIN, acute interstitial nephritis; AKI, acute kidney injury; ARB, angiotensin receptor blockers; ATN, acute tubular necrosis; BUN, blood urea nitrogen; CHF, congestive heart failure; Cr, creatinine; DM, diabetes mellitus; FENa, fractional excretion of sodium; NSAID, nonsteroidal anti-inflammatory drugs; PCTA, percutaneous transluminal coronary angioplasty; TLS, tumor lysis syndrome; UTI, urinary tract infection.
   Data from Refs.[31,63,64]

or excess use of diuretics. Other specified risk factors for hospital-acquired AKI are outlined in **Fig. 7**.[66,67]

Sepsis

AKI is common in the ICU setting with occurrences as high as 65%, with mortality rates approaching 30%.[9,12] The pathophysiology of AKI in sepsis is complex and

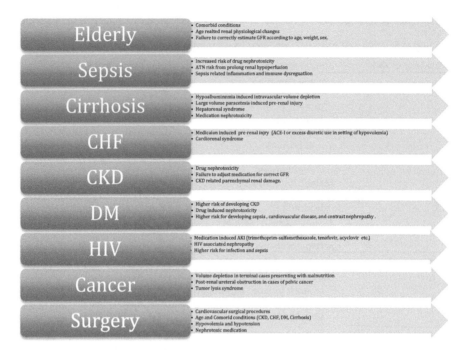

Fig. 6. Specific patients at risk for hospital acquired acute kidney injury (AKI). ACE-I, angiotensin converting enzyme inhibitors; CHF, congestive heart failure; CKD, chronic kidney disease; DM, Diabetes mellitus; HIV, human immunodeficiency virus. (*Data from* Refs.[23,37,67,68,71,74,75])

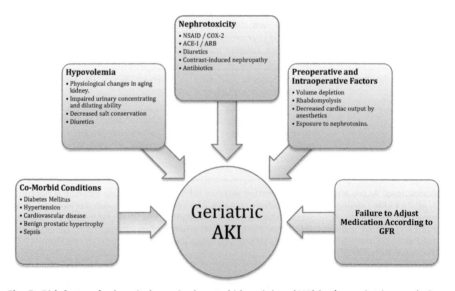

Fig. 7. Risk factors for hospital acquired acute kidney injury (AKI) in the geriatric population. ACE-I, angiotensin converting enzyme inhibitors; ARB, Angiotensin receptor blockers; COX-2, cyclooxygenase 2 inhibitors; GFR, glomerular filtration rate; NSAID, Nonsteroidal anti-inflammatory drugs. (*Data from* Chronopoulos A, Cruz DN, Ronco C. Hospital-acquired acute kidney injury in the elderly. Nat Rev Nephrol 2010;6:141–49; and Abdel-Kader K, Palevsky P. Acute kidney injury in the elderly. Clin Geriatr Med 2009;25(3):331–58.)

multifactorial including renal hypoperfusion causing ischemic ATN, nephrotoxic medication exposure, and sepsis-induced endothelial dysfunction with infiltration of inflammatory cells in renal parenchyma.[68] Furthermore, development of AKI in setting of sepsis is associated with greater mortality and risk for developing permanent renal failure requiring renal replacement therapy.[9,68,69]

Cirrhosis

In the hospital setting, it is important to appreciate that patients with advanced cirrhosis will have low creatinine production because of reduced muscle mass, leading to lower serum creatinine laboratory values. This circumstance can falsely overestimate a patient's true GFR, which can lead clinicians to underestimate the risk for developing AKI.

Cirrhotic patients are highly prone to pre-renal injury from intravascular volume depletion secondary to gastrointestinal bleeding, diuretic use, and lactulose-induced diarrhea. Also, because albumin is exclusively synthesized in liver, lower albumin production often predisposes such patients to higher incidences of pre-renal injury from reduced effective arterial blood volume, especially after undergoing large volume paracentesis.[38] ATN in cirrhosis is also commonly owing to medication nephrotoxicity, sepsis, and IV contrast agents.

The hepatorenal syndrome is a devastating disease afflicting patients with decompensated cirrhosis and is associated with high in-hospital mortality approaching 50% within 1 month of diagnosis. Advanced portal hypertension causes profuse systemic arterial vasodilatation, with prolonged renal hypoperfusion resulting in severe AKI. Diagnostic considerations include[37,38]:

- Serum creatinine greater than 1.5 mg/dL (133 μmol/L);
- No improvement in serum creatinine after at least 2 days of diuretic withdrawal and expansion of plasma volume with albumin;
- No current or recent treatment with nephrotoxic drugs or vasodilators; and
- Fractional excretion of sodium (FENa) of less than 1%.

Treatment modalities include administration of IV albumin in conjunction with the vasoconstrictors, such as midodrine, but prognosis remains guarded.[37,38]

Chronic Kidney Disease

Patients afflicted with CKD often have increased comorbidities including DM, CHF, and hypertension that require treatment with ACE-I and diuretics that increase the risk of pre-renal disease in the setting of acute volume depletion or hypovolemia.[40,70,71] Furthermore, advanced CKD patients have structural parenchymal damage, including tubular hypertrophy, interstitial fibrosis, and a variable degree of glomerulosclerosis. Collectively, these changes can predispose CKD patients to impaired autoregulation of renal blood flow and AKI, especially with regard to drug nephrotoxicity and CIN.[70,71] To further complicate matters, CKD patients with AKI are less likely to recover renal function, and have an increased risk of developing end-stage renal disease.[72]

Human Immunodeficiency Virus Infection

Compared with noninfected hospitalized patients, AKI was documented in a significantly greater proportion of HIV-infected hospitalized patients. Advanced age (>65 year), DM, preexisting CKD, and chronic liver disease with hepatitis C are specific patient-related risk factors in this population.[73,74] ATN from nephrotoxic medication such as tenofovir, or AIN from trimethoprim-sulfamethoxazole and acyclovir remain common causes of AKI (see **Table 1**).

HIV nephropathy is the most common glomerular disease in patients with advanced or poorly controlled disease. Clinical presentation includes renal failure with significant proteinuria, often in the setting of normal blood pressure and normal to enlarged kidneys.[73,74]

Perioperative Acute Kidney Injury

Perioperative AKI is common in the hospital setting with estimated prevalence of 30% to 40%. The development of perioperative AKI has been independently linked with worse patient outcomes, including increased morbidity such as AKI requiring dialysis initiation and mortality.[75,76] Patients undergoing cardiac, vascular, and major abdominal surgery are at greatest risk for developing AKI. Pre-renal and ischemic ATN are the most common causes of AKI in this setting. Multiple risk factors, including older age, CKD, CHF, sepsis, liver failure, and concurrent use of nephrotoxic agents predispose patients to perioperative AKI.[75,76]

Intraoperative AKI risk factors often include hypovolemia and ischemic AKI from prolonged hypotension, cardiopulmonary bypass time during cardiac surgery, aortic cross-clamp time during vascular procedures, and duration of surgery. Rhabdomyolysis is also an important cause of intraoperative AKI as a result of extended periods of immobilization, related to intraoperative patient positioning. Other risk factors include concurrent use of nephrotoxic medication and use of imaging with IV iodinated contrast.[75,76]

CLINICAL EVALUATION OF ACUTE KIDNEY INJURY IN THE HOSPITAL SETTING

The clinical evaluation of AKI should begin with early recognition of increases in serum creatinine or alterations in GFR as seen in RIFLE criteria (see **Fig. 1**). Categorization of AKI will also help to narrow differential diagnosis responsible for the acute renal insult (see **Fig. 2**).

History and Clinical Evaluation

Patients who develop AKI in the hospital setting usually have an identifiable initiating event that can be found from review of vital signs, laboratory data, urine output records, and medications. A past medical history should focus on evaluation for medical conditions at higher risk for AKI (see **Fig. 6**). Review of past medical records including outpatient laboratory results can determine if there is any prior history of impaired renal function. Particular attention should be made in investigating how well comorbid conditions such as diabetes, hypertension, CHF, and HIV have been managed in the outpatient setting. Concurrent sepsis and gastrointestinal losses, such as diarrhea, nausea, vomiting, or changes in appetite suggested by weight loss can help to establish important risk factors for pre-renal AKI. Review of hospital and outpatient records should also focus on medications, herbal remedies, vitamins, and analgesics as well as any recent diagnostic imaging with contrast. Previous documented allergies, especially antibiotics, may help in diagnosing cases of AIN.

Physical examination should focus on vital signs, including fever, changes in blood pressure, and urine output measurements during hospitalization. Clinicians should use judgment to carefully monitor a patient's hemodynamic status in the hospital setting, especially with regard to blood pressure medication dose adjustments, to avoid hypotension. This is most problematic in acutely ill patients who are admitted with hypovolemia and medicated with ACE-I, ARB, or NSAIDs, which can further reduce renal perfusion pressures with a subsequent greater risk of developing AKI. To avoid AKI, their blood pressure dosing regimens should be monitored closely with hold parameters to avoid hypotension. Furthermore, in the setting of acute illness, even minor reductions in systolic blood pressure, 14 mm Hg or greater, termed relative hypotension, has been attributed to cause AKI.[77]

Evaluating acute changes in urine output has important prognostic implications for the severity of AKI as seen by classification of RIFLE criteria.[4–6,10] Oliguria is defined as reduction in urine output of less than 500 mL/d, and anuria as less than 50 mL. Furthermore, oliguric ATN has been associated with increased risk of mortality and requirement for renal replacement therapy in comparison to nonoliguric AKI conditions.[78,79]

Patients with acute onset of oliguria without risk factors for pre-renal or intrinsic disease should be evaluated for post-renal AKI. Clinical risk factors for obstructive uropathy include BPH, prostate cancer, and pelvic tumors. Neurogenic bladder is a dysfunction of the urinary bladder owing to diseases of the central nervous system or peripheral nerves involved in the control of micturition. Patient risk factors include advanced DM, spinal cord disease such as paraplegia, or cerebrovascular accident. A simple bedside evaluation should include a bladder ultrasound scan to assess post void residual bladder volume. Any value greater than 100 mL is suggestive of bladder outlet obstruction. Renal ultrasonography or noncontrast CT imaging can help to evaluate upper urinary tract obstructions such as nephrolithiasis.[61,62]

Laboratory Data

Common laboratory and urine results used to help differentiate among different category of AKI are outlined in **Table 2**. Serum creatinine and blood urea nitrogen are the usual starting points for the evaluation of AKI. Urea is a byproduct of protein metabolism and can also be elevated in cases of gastrointestinal bleeding and with medications such as steroids. The blood urea nitrogen to serum creatinine ratio is often greater than 20:1 in pre-renal disease owing to the increase in the passive reabsorption of urea that follows the enhanced proximal reabsorption of sodium and water (see **Table 2**).[31,63] As mentioned, creatinine generation varies according to individual patient factors such as age, sex, gender, and muscle mass. Therefore, creatinine measurements, in itself, may not always be an accurate depiction of a patient's true estimated GFR.[2,21]

Serum cystatin C has been shown to be more sensitive and rapid means to detect AKI compared with serum creatinine. Combining both the serum creatinine and cystatin C into a single equation may better estimate GFR. However, its current use in hospital setting is limited owing to high cost and ongoing investigational trials will help to determine its clinical impact on patient outcomes in the future.[80,81]

Examination of urine studies is helpful in categorizing causes of AKI. Urinalysis should focus on determination of specific gravity, presence of proteinuria and red blood cells in glomerular injury or white blood cells in cases of interstitial damage.[31,54,63] Microscopic examination of the urine may show sediments such as coarse granular casts in ATN or dysmorphic red blood cell casts in cases of acute glomerulonephritis. Urine chemistries such as spot concentrations of urine sodium and creatinine can be used to calculate the FENa. The FENa is calculated as the ratio of urine to plasma sodium concentration divided by urine to plasma creatinine concentrations. This calculation can help in differentiating pre-renal disease from ATN. In general, a FENa of less than 1% suggests pre-renal disease. A relatively high FENa of greater than 2% is more indicative of ATN, demonstrating inappropriate sodium wasting because of tubular damage. Use of diuretics reduces the utility of FENa. An alternative is to calculate the fractional excretion of urea, defined as the ratio of urine to plasma urea concentration divided by urine to plasma creatinine concentrations.[31,54,63]

Glomerular disease can be caused by primary or secondary etiologies. Family history of CKD and comorbid conditions can help to identify potential secondary causes that commonly lead to glomerular damage (see **Fig. 5**).[54] Secondary workup should include specific diagnostic laboratory evaluations (**Table 3**). Random protein to creatinine ratio and 24-hour collection of urine protein will help to differentiate nephritic versus non-nephrotic proteinuria. Urine protein electrophoresis and serum protein electrophoresis can help to evaluate for monoclonal gammopathies such as multiple myeloma or amyloidosis.

RADIOGRAPHIC IMAGING AND DIAGNOSTIC PROCEDURES

Renal and bladder ultrasonography should be performed on all patients with AKI. In particular, these imaging modalities can help to evaluate for obstructive uropathy. A bladder residual volume of greater than 100 mL (determined by bladder scan) is suggestive of bladder outlet obstruction, especially in geriatric patients who have history of BPH or at risk for neurogenic bladder. CT without contrast is the preferred diagnostic modality in cases of AKI attributed to complex nephrolithiasis or retroperitoneal tumors as in cases of complex nephrolithiasis or retroperitoneal tumors.[61]

Renal biopsy is helpful in cases where diagnostic confirmation of renal pathology is required before initiation of immune-modulating therapies, particularly nephritic and nephritic syndromes (see **Fig. 5**). Laboratory investigations should be done before performing a renal biopsy to help pathologist narrow the differential diagnosis for AKI (see **Table 3**). In cases where a renal biopsy is being contemplated, a nephrologist should be consulted to review the case and discuss important risks and benefits of the procedure. Some relative contraindications for renal biopsy include active infection, small atrophic kidneys, solitary native kidney, hydronephrosis, severe hypertension, and conditions causing coagulopathy or thrombocytopenia that increases the risk of bleeding.[54]

Table 3	
Laboratory diagnosis of glomerular diseases	
Laboratory Test	**Suggestive Glomerular Disease**
Serum ANA and Anti-ds DNA	Lupus nephritis (SLE)
Low complements (C3, C4)	Lupus nephritis, postinfectious glomerulosclerosis (post-streptococcal and endocarditis), hepatitis C–associated membranoproliferative glomerulonephritis and cryoglobulinemia
Antiglomerular basement antibody	Rapidly progressive glomerulonephritis (Goodpasture syndrome)
Antineutrophilic cytoplasmic antibody	Rapidly progressive glomerulonephritis (Wegeners syndrome).
Cryoglobulin	Cryoglobulinemia especially in cases of Hepatitis C
HIV	Collapsing focal segmental glomerulosclerosis
SPEP and UPEP	Monoclonal gammopathies: Amyloidosis and multiple myeloma

Abbreviations: ANA, anti-nuclear antibody; anti-ds DNA, anti-double stranded DNA; HIV, human immunodeficiency virus; SLE, systemic lupus erythematosis; SPEP, serum protein electropharesis; UPEP, urine protein electropharesis.

Data from Hricik D, Chung-Park M, Sedor JR. Glomerulonephritis. N Engl J Med 1998;339:888–99; and Floege J, Feehally J. Introduction to glomerular disease: clinical presentations. In: Floege J, Johnson RJ, Feehally J, editors. Comprehensive clinical nephrology. 4th edition. Philadelphia: WB Saunders; 2010. p. 193–207.

TREATMENT AND PREVENTION

Treatment of AKI entails prompt identification of AKI, as outlined by the RIFLE classification (see **Fig. 1**), while making an effort to categorize AKI according to an appropriate category (see **Fig. 2**). It is critical to first classify AKI as either non-oliguric or oliguric, with the oliguric AKI having worse clinical outcomes associated with more serious metabolic and volume disturbances.[79] Clinicians should also recognize that AKI is associated with severe electrolytes abnormalities, such as hyperkalemia and metabolic acidosis, which can cause fatal cardiac arrhythmias. Important treatment goals for hospital-acquired AKI are also outlined in **Box 1** and **Table 4**.

Despite high mortality rates associated with AKI, most conventional therapies are aimed at treating the underlying conditions that cause the acute insult, rather than at the kidneys themselves. Clinical trials have failed to show any success with the use of agents, such as dopamine agonists, furosemide, fenoldopam, and atrial natriuretic peptide analogs in the treatment of AKI.[43]

Pre-renal

The goal in pre-renal AKI is to normalize renal perfusion pressures by administration of IV fluids, such as isotonic saline, while holding diuretics, NSAIDs, and blood pressure

---

Box 1
Prevention and treatment of contrast-induced nephropathy

Use lowest osmolar contrast agents (avoid high osmolar agents [>900 mosmol/kg]).

Use lower doses of IV contrast and avoid repetitive studies.

Before administration of IV contrast, ensure that the patient is not volume depleted.

• Avoid concurrent use of NSAIDs.

• If possible, temporarily hold ACE-I or ARB medication before and immediately after contrast.

If there is no contraindication to volume expansion, for example, CHF, administer either normal saline or isotonic bicarbonate for 6 to12 hours before and after IV contrast:

• Normal saline (0.9%) IV at 1 mL/kg per hour, begun at least 6 to 12 hours before the procedure, and continued 6 to 12 hours after contrast procedure; or

• 150 mEq of sodium bicarbonate in D5W IV at 3 mL/kg per hour for 1 hour before and 1 mL/kg per hour for 6 hours after procedure.

Concurrent use of NAC at 1200 mg orally twice daily 1 day before and after the day of the contrast procedure.

• Despite conflicting data, NAC seems to be safe and inexpensive with potential prophylactic benefits.

Avoid magnetic resonance imaging gadolinium imaging in unstable patients with new onset of AKI or advanced CKD with of GFR less than 30.

Abbreviations: ACE-I, angiotensin converting enzyme inhibitors; AKI, acute kidney injury; ARB, angiotensin receptor blockers; CKD, chronic kidney disease; D5W, dextrose with 5% water; GFR, glomerular filtration rate; IV, intravenous; NAC, *N*-acetylcysteine; NSAID, nonsteroidal anti-inflammatory drugs.

Data from Refs.[43,45,82]

medications that can contribute to pre-renal AKI. Patients with decompensated heart failure can also have pre-renal urine indices including low urinary sodium and FENa. However, instead of IV fluids, these patients will require aggressive use of diuretics and possibly inotropic agents to improve renal perfusion.[39]

Table 4
Treatment goals for hospital-acquired AKI

Category of AKI	Treatment Goals
Pre-renal	• Optimize hemodynamic status to achieve euvolemia with isotonic fluid administration. • Stop ACE-I/ARB/NSAID if hypovolemic or hypotensive. • Adjust antihypertensive medications to avoid hypotension. • If gastrointestinal losses; treat underlying causes. • Treat electrolyte disorders (hyperkalemia, metabolic acidosis, hyponatremia, hypernatremia).
ATN	• Treat any ongoing pre-renal insult, eg, sepsis, gastrointestinal losses or causes of hypotension. • Discontinue any nephrotoxic medications (see Table 1). • Avoid any IV contrast imaging unless emergently needed. • Make dose adjustments in medication according to estimated GFR. • If trauma or history of fall, evaluate for rhabdomyolysis. • If recent surgery done, evaluate anesthesia reports, medications, vitals. • If oliguric, evaluate ultrasound of kidneys and bladder scan. • If oliguric with refractory life threatening hyperkalemia and/or metabolic acidosis that fails to be treated with conservative therapy, consider renal replacement therapy.
AIN	• Evaluate clinically for acute drug rash and allergy history. • Rule out possible causes of pre-renal and ATN. • Evaluate if any causal relationship between medication start and development of AKI (see Table 1). • Evaluate for urine eosinophils and peripheral eosinophilia.
Glomerular	• Evaluate any comorbid conditions at risk for glomerular disease (see Fig. 5). • Check serologic studies for glomerular diseases (see Table 3). • Consider renal biopsy if no contraindications in cases of nephritic or nephrotic diseases if approved by nephrologist. • Tailor immunosuppressive medication based on renal biopsy result including possible steroids, immunotherapy, and in cases of RPGN or TTP, consider plasma exchange if approved by nephrologist.
Post-renal	• Prompt placement of bladder foley catheter if oliguric or urinary retention. • Start with bladder and renal ultrasound to evaluate for obstructive uropathy and hydronephrosis. • If history of nephrolithiasis or pelvic cancer, evaluate with CT non-contrast imaging. • Initiate BPH medications for enlarged prostate. • Evaluate for offending medications that can cause urinary retention. • If complex nephrolithiasis or prostate disease, consult urology for surgical intervention.

Abbreviations: ACE-I, angiotensin converting enzyme inhibitors; AIN, acute interstitial nephritis; ARB, angiotensin receptor blockers; ATN, acute tubular necrosis; BPH, benign prostatic hypertrophy; CT, computed tomography; GFR, glomerular filtration rate; NSAID, Nonsteroidal anti-inflammatory drugs; RPGN, rapidly progressive glomerulonephritis; TTP, thrombotic thrombocytopenic purpura.
Data from Refs.[31,43,54]

Acute Tubular Necrosis

Beside supportive care and treatment of underlying medical conditions, no specific therapeutic agent has been shown to treat ATN. Preventative measures for CIN are outlined in **Box 1**.[43,45,82]

The first priority should be aimed at evaluating urine output, volume status, and recognizing potential nephrotoxic medications. Nonoliguric ATN is associated with better prognosis and renal recovery.[31,79] Oliguric patients with refractory hyperkalemia and severe metabolic acidosis or volume overload that fail to be treated with medical therapy may require initiation of renal replacement therapy, especially in the setting of rhabdomyolysis or sepsis.[31,78]

Acute Interstitial Nephritis

Most cases of AIN owing to drugs improve within several days to weeks after the discontinuation of the offending medication. In severe cases, oral glucocorticoids may have some benefit in improving renal outcomes.[28,52] If the patient experiences AIN in the hospital setting, the allergic reaction should be permanently documented in the patient's hospital record to avoid recurrent AKI on future admissions.

Glomerular and Vascular Damage

Rapidly progressive glomerulonephritis and TTP are 2 serious causes of glomerular damage associated with permanent renal injury. In the case of TTP, prompt initiation of plasma exchange will help to avoid systemic thrombosis and ischemic damage. Wegners and Goodpastures syndromes also require initiation of immunosuppressive medication, such as cyclophosphamide, combined with high-dose IV glucocorticoids. In severe cases, plasma exchange will also help to improve patient outcomes.[83]

Patients with endocarditis or bacteremia can present with postinfectious glomerulonephritis; treatment entails prolonged antibiotics to eradicate infection. Systemic lupus erythematosus can also lead to severe proliferative glomerular damage with

Table 5
Medication associated with urinary retention

Class of Medication	Medication
Anticholinergics	Atropine, oxybutynin, scopolamine.
Antidepressants	Amitriptyline, imipramine, nortriptyline.
Antihistamines	Diphenhydramine, hydroxyzine, brompheniramine.
Parkinson Treatment	Amantadine, benztropine mesylate, bromocriptine, levodopa, trihexyphenidyl.
Antipsychotics	Chlorpromazine, haloperidol, prochlorperazine.
Muscle relaxants	Baclofen, cyclobenzaprine, diazepam
Sympathomimetics (α-adrenergic agents)	Ephedrine, phenylephrine, pseudoephedrine.
Sympathomimetics (β-adrenergic agents)	Isoproterenol, terbutaline.

Data from Curtis LA, Dolan TS, Cespedes RD. Acute urinary retention and urinary incontinence. Emerg Med Clin North Am 2001;19(3):591–619; and Frokiaer J, Zeidel M. Urinary tract obstruction. In: Taal MW, Chertow GM, Marsden PA, et al, editors. Brenner and Rector's the kidney. 9th edition. New York: Elsevier; 2011.

the development of AKI and is often treated with high-dose glucocorticoids and immunosuppressive medications.

Post-renal

Treatment is based on identifying the anatomic location of the lower or upper urinary tract obstruction and placement of a bladder catheter in cases of AKI. Lower tract obstructions are commonly caused by BPH, neurogenic bladder, or medications that inhibit bladder contraction. Initiation of medication such as selective α-blockers or 5-α reductase inhibitors will help in the management of BPH. A urology consult may be needed in cases of advanced BPH or prostate cancer that require chronic bladder catheter use. In cases of urinary retention, any offending medications should be discontinued (**Table 5**). Cases of upper urinary tract obstruction, such as nephrolithiasis causing hydronephrosis, may require urologic intervention with ureteral stent placement in severe cases.

SUMMARY

AKI is becoming an increasingly common problem in the hospital setting, especially among elderly and ICU populations, and is independently associated with an increased mortality and risk for development of permanent CKD. Prevention of hospital acquired AKI is important and standardized definitions have evolved, such as the RIFLE criteria, which have led to heightened awareness for early diagnosis of acute renal injury. Proper diagnosis and treatment of AKI requires clinicians to understand the basic classifications of AKI, such as pre-renal, intrinsic, and post-renal, while investigating important causative factors for each of the categories. Accordingly, clinicians should also identify patient populations at higher risk for developing AKI while making efforts to avoid iatrogenic insults, such as nephrotoxic medications and IV radiocontrast imaging when appropriate.

REFERENCES

1. Bellomo R, Kellum JA, Ronco C. Acute kidney injury. Lancet 2012;380:756–66.
2. Thadhani R, Pascual M, Bonventre JV. Acute renal failure. N Engl J Med 1996; 344:1448–60.
3. Bellomo R, Kellum JA, Ronco C, et al. Acute renal failure – definition, outcome measures, animal models, fluid therapy, and information technology needs: the second international consensus of the Acute Dialysis Quality Initiative (ADQI) group. Crit Care 2004;8:R204–12.
4. Hoste E, Schurgers M. Epidemiology of acute kidney injury: how big is the problem? Crit Care Med 2008;36(4):S146–51.
5. Wang HE, Muntner P, Chertow GM, et al. Acute kidney injury and mortality in hospitalized patients. Am J Nephrol 2012;35:349–55.
6. Chertow GM, Burdick E, Honour M, et al. Acute kidney injury, mortality, length of stay, and costs in hospitalized patients. J Am Soc Nephrol 2005;16:3365–70.
7. Liangos O, Wald R, O'Bell JW, et al. Epidemiology and outcomes of acute renal failure in hospitalized patients: a national survey. Clin J Am Soc Nephrol 2006;1: 43–51.
8. Singbart K, Kellum JA. AKI in the ICU: definition, epidemiology, risk stratification, and outcomes. Kidney Int 2012;81:819–25.
9. Hoste EA, Clermont G, Kersten A, et al. RIFLE criteria for acute kidney injury are associated with hospital mortality in critically ill patients: a cohort analysis. Crit Care 2006;10(3):R73.

10. Meran S, Wonnacott A, Amphlett B, et al. How good are we at managing acute kidney injury in hospital? Clin Kidney J 2014;7(2):144–50.

11. Case J, Khan S, Khalid R, et al. Epidemiology of acute kidney injury in the intensive care unit. Crit Care Res Pract 2013;2013:479730.

12. Ricci Z, Cruz D, Ronco C. The RIFLE criteria and mortality in acute kidney injury: a systemic review. Kidney Int 2008;73:538–46.

13. Uchino S, Bellomo R, Goldsmith D, et al. An assessment of the RIFLE criteria for acute renal failure in hospitalized patients. Crit Care 2006;34(7):1913–7.

14. Matzke GR, Aronoff GR, Atinson AJ, et al. Drug dosing consideration in patients with acute and chronic kidney disease- a clinical update from Kidney disease: Improving Globe Outcomes (KDIGO). Kidney Int 2011;80:1122–37.

15. Hudson JQ, Nyman HA. Use of estimated glomerular filtration rate for drug dosing in the chronic kidney disease patient. Curr Opin Nephrol Hypertens 2011;20(5):482–91.

16. Perrone RD, Madias NE, Levey AS. Serum creatinine as an index of renal function: new insights into old concepts. Clin Chem 1992;38:1933–53.

17. Waikar S, Bonventre JV. Creatinine kinetics and the definition of acute kidney injury. J Am Soc Nephrol 2009;20(3):672–9.

18. Traynor J, Mactier R, Geddes C, et al. How to measure renal function in clinical practice. BMJ 2006;333(7571):733–7.

19. Poggio ED, Nef PC, Wang X, et al. Performance of the Cockcroft-Gault and modification of diet in renal disease equations in estimating GFR in ill hospitalized patients. Am J Kidney Dis 2005;46(2):242–52.

20. Bragadottir G, Redfors B, Ricksten SE. Assessing glomerular filtration rate (GFR) in critically ill patients with acute kidney injury- true GFR versus urinary creatinine clearance and estimating equations. Crit Care 2013;17:R108.

21. Stevens LA, Coresh J, Greene T, et al. Assessing kidney function-measured and estimated glomerular filtration rate. N Engl J Med 2006; 354:2473–83.

22. Liano F, Pascual J. Epidemiology of acute renal failure: a prospective, multicenter, community-based study. Madrid acute renal failure study group. Kidney Int 1996;50:811–8.

23. Nolan C, Anderson R. Hospital acquired acute renal failure. J Am Soc Nephrol 1998;9:710–8.

24. Perazella M. Toxic nephropathies: core curriculum 2010. Am J Kidney Dis 2010; 55(2):399–409.

25. Nally JV. Acute renal failure in hospitalized patients. Cleve Clin J Med 2002; 69(7):569–74.

26. Schetz M, Dasta J, Goldstein S, et al. Drug-induced acute kidney injury. Curr Opin Crit Care 2005;11:555–65.

27. Guo X, Nzerue C. How to prevent, recognize, and treat drug-induced nephrotoxicity. Cleve Clin J Med 2002;69(4):289–312.

28. Praga M, Gonzalez E. Acute interstitial nephritis. Kidney Int 2010;77:956–61.

29. Perazella MA. Renal vulnerability to drug toxicity. Clin J Am Soc Nephrol 2009;4: 1275–83.

30. Lameire N. The pathophysiology of acute renal failure. Crit Care Clin 2005;21: 197–210.

31. Macedo E, Mehta RL. Epidemiology, diagnosis, and therapy of acute kidney injury. In: Coffman TM, Falk RJ, Molitoris BA, et al, editors. Schrier's diseases of the kidney. 9th edition. Philadelphia: Lippincott Williams & Wilkins; 2013. p. 785–825.

32. Tomlinson LA, Abel GA, Chaudhry AN, et al. ACE inhibitor and angiotensin receptor-II antagonist prescribing and hospital admissions with acute kidney injury: a longitudinal ecological study. PLoS One 2013;8(11):e78465.

33. Schoolwerth AC, Sica DA, Ballermann BJ, et al. Renal consideration in angiotensin converting enzyme inhibitor therapy. Circulation 2001;104:1985–91.

34. Whelton A. Nephrotoxicity of nonsteroidal anti-inflammatory drugs: physiologic foundations and clinical implications. Am J Med 1999;106:13S–24S.

35. Perazella MA, Tray K. Selective cyclooxygenase-2 inhibitors: a patter of nephrotoxicity similar to traditional nonsteroidal anti-inflammatory drugs. Am J Med 2001;111:64–71.

36. Palmer B. Nephrotoxicity of nonsteroidal anti-inflammatory agents, analgesics, and inhibitors of the rennin-angiotensin system. In: Coffman TM, Falk RJ, Molitoris BA, et al, editors. Schrier's diseases of the kidney. 9th edition. Philadelphia: Lippincott Williams & Wilkins; 2013. p. 943–58.

37. Gines P, Schrier RW. Renal failure in cirrhosis. N Engl J Med 2009;361:1279–90.

38. Wadei HM, Mai ML, Ahsan N, et al. Hepatorenal syndrome: pathophysiology and management. Clin J Am Soc Nephrol 2006;1:1066–79.

39. Ronco C, Haapio M, House AA, et al. Cardiorenal syndrome. J Am Coll Cardiol 2008;52:1527–39.

40. Girman CJ, Kou TD, Brodovicz K, et al. Risk of acute renal failure with type 2 diabetes mellitus. Diabet Med 2012;29(5):614–21.

41. Barrett BJ. Contrast nephrotoxicity. J Am Soc Nephrol 1994;5:125–37.

42. Rudnick MR, Kesselheim A, Goldfarb S. Contrast-induced nephropathy: how it develops, how to prevent it. Cleve Clin J Med 2006;73(1):75–87.

43. Eckardt KU, Kasiske B, Kellum JA, et al. Kidney Disease: Improving Global Outcomes (KDIGO) Acute Kidney Injury Work Group. KDIGO Clinical Practice Guideline for Acute Kidney Injury. Kidney Inter 2012;2(Suppl):1–138.

44. Deo A, Fogel M, Cowper SE. Nephrogenic systemic fibrosis: a population study examining the relationship of disease development to gadolinium exposure. Clin J Am Soc Nephrol 2007;2(2):264–7.

45. Perazella M. Gadolinium-contrast toxicity in patients with kidney disease: nephrotoxicity and nephrogenic systemic fibrosis. Curr Drug Saf 2008;3:67–75.

46. Vanholder R, Sever MS, Erek E, et al. Rhabdomyolysis. J Am Soc Nephrol 2000; 11(8):1553–61.

47. Bosch X, Poch E, Grau JM. Rhabdomyolysis and acute kidney injury. N Engl J Med 2009;361:62–72.

48. Howard SC, Jones DP, Pui CH. The tumor lysis syndrome. N Engl J Med 2011; 364:1844–54.

49. Rossert J. Drug induced acute interstitial nephritis. Kidney Int 2001;60:804–17.

50. Perazella MA, Markowitz GS. Drug induced acute interstitial nephritis. Nat Rev Nephrol 2010;6:461–70.

51. Muriithi AK, Nasr SH, Leung N. Utility of urine eosinophils in the diagnosis of acute interstitial nephritis. Clin J Am Soc Nephrol 2013;8(11):1857–62.

52. Gonzales E, Gutierrez E, Galeano C, et al. Early steroid treatment improves the recovery of renal function in patients with drug-induced acute interstitial nephritis. Kidney Int 2008;73:940–6.

53. Hricik D, Chung-Park M, Sedor JR. Glomerulonephritis. N Engl J Med 1998;339: 888–99.

54. Floege J, Feehally J. Introduction to glomerular disease: clinical presentations. In: Floege J, Johnson RJ, Feehally J, editors. Comprehensive clinical nephrology. 4th edition. Philadelphia: WB Saunders; 2010. p. 193–207.

55. Jennette JC. Rapidly progressive crescentic glomerulonephritis. Kidney Int 2003;63:1164–77.
56. Nasr SH, Radhakrishnan J, D'Agati VD. Bacterial infection-related glomerulonephritis in adults. Kidney Int 2013;83:792–803.
57. Scolari F, Ravani P. Atheroembolic renal disease. Lancet 2010;375:1650–60.
58. Ruggenenti P, Noris M, Remuzzi G. Thrombotic microangiopathy, hemolytic uremic syndrome, and thrombotic thrombocytopenia purpura. Kidney Int 2001;60: 831–46.
59. Moake JL. Thrombotic microangiopathies. N Engl J Med 2002;347:589–600.
60. George JN. How I treat patients with thrombotic thrombocytopenia purpura: 2010. Blood 2010;116(20):4060–9.
61. Frokiaer J, Zeidel M. Urinary tract obstruction. In: Taal MW, Chertow GM, Marsden PA, et al, editors. Brenner and Rector's the kidney. 9th edition. New York: Elsevier; 2011. p. 1239–64.
62. Curtis LA, Dolan TS, Cespedes RD. Acute urinary retention and urinary incontinence. Emerg Med Clin North Am 2001;19(3):591–619.
63. Schrier RW, Wang W, Poole B, et al. Acute renal failure: definitions, diagnosis, pathogenesis, and therapy. J Clin Invest 2004;114:5–14.
64. Yang L, Bonventre JV. Diagnosis and clinical evaluation of acute kidney injury. In: Floege J, Johnson RJ, Feehally J, editors. Comprehensive clinical nephrology. 4th edition. Philadelphia: WB Saunders; 2010. p. 821–9.
65. United States Renal Data System (USRDS). Data report on acute kidney injury. Chapter 6. 2013. Available at: http://www.usrds.org/2013/view/v1_06.aspx. Accessed on January 10, 2014.
66. Abdel-Kader K, Palevsky P. Acute kidney injury in the elderly. Clin Geriatr Med 2009;25(3):331–58.
67. Chronopoulos A, Cruz DN, Ronco C. Hospital-acquired acute kidney injury in the elderly. Nat Rev Nephrol 2010;6:141–9.
68. Zarjou A, Agarwal A. Sepsis and acute kidney injury. J Am Soc Nephrol 2011; 22(6):999–1006.
69. Ronco C, Kellum JA, Bellomo R, et al. Potential interventions in sepsis related AKI. Clin J Am Soc Nephrol 2008;3(2):531–44.
70. Thakar CV, Christianson A, Himmelfarb J, et al. Chronic kidney disease risk in diabetes mellitus. Clin J Am Soc Nephrol 2011;6(1):2567–72.
71. Chawla LS, Kimmel PL. Acute kidney injury and chronic kidney disease: an integrated clinical syndrome. Kidney Int 2012;82:516–24.
72. Ishani A, Xue JL, Himmelfarb J, et al. Acute kidney injury increases risk of ESRD among elderly. J Am Soc Nephrol 2009;20:223–38.
73. Franceschini N, Napravnik S, Eron JJ, et al. Incidence and etiology of acute renal failure among ambulatory HIV-infected patients. Kidney Int 2005;67(4): 1526–31.
74. Wyatt CM, Arons RR, Klotman PE, et al. Acute renal failure in hospitalized patients with HIV: risk factors and impact on in-hospital mortality. AIDS 2006; 20(4):561–5.
75. Thakar CV. Perioperative acute kidney injury. Adv Chronic Kidney Dis 2013; 20(1):561–5.
76. Borthwick E, Ferguson A. Perioperative acute kidney injury: risk factors, recognition, management, and outcomes. BMJ 2010;341:85–91.
77. Liu YL, Prowle J, Licari E, et al. Changes in blood pressure before the development of nosocomial acute kidney injury. Nephrol Dial Transplant 2009;24: 504–11.

78. Mandelbaum T, Lee J, Scott DJ, et al. Empirical relationships among oliguria, creatinine, mortality, and renal replacement therapy in the critically ill. Intensive Care Med 2013;39(3):414–9.

79. Oh HJ, Shin DH, Lee MJ, et al. Urine output is associated with prognosis in patients with acute kidney injury requiring continuous renal replacement therapy. J Crit Care 2013;28(4):379–88.

80. Inker LA, Schmid CH, Tighiouart H, et al. Estimating glomerular filtration rate from serum creatinine and cystatin C. N Engl J Med 2012;367:20–9.

81. Zhang Z, Lu B, Sheng X, et al. Cystatin C in prediction of acute kidney injury: a systemic review and meta-analysis. Am J Kidney Dis 2011;58(3):356–65.

82. Rim MY, Ro H, Kang WC, et al. The effect of rennin-angiotensin-aldosterone system blockade on contrast-induced acute kidney injury: a propensity matched study. Am J Kidney Dis 2012;60(4):576–82.

83. Pusey CD, Levy JB. Plasmapharesis in immunologic renal disease. Blood Purif 2012;33(1–3):190–8.

Nonsteroidal Antiinflammatory Drugs, Cyclooxygenase-2, and the Kidneys

Saadur Rahman, DO[a], Anthony Malcoun, DO[b,c],*

KEYWORDS

- NSAIDS • COX-1 • COX-2 • Kidneys • Hypertension • Acute kidney injury
- Electrolytes • Glomerular filtration rate

KEY POINTS

- Nonsteroidal antiinflammatory drugs (NSAIDs) are the most commonly prescribed medications, and about 2.5 million people in the United States will experience NSAID-mediated renal disease.
- NSAIDs can cause acute kidney injury from glomerular hypoperfusion, especially in the setting of intravascular volume depletion, or concomitant use of medications that can alter renal autoregulation, such as angiotensin-converting enzyme inhibitors and angiotensin receptor blockers.
- Acute interstitial nephritis is a well-known side effect of NSAIDs, and its preferred treatment is immediate cessation of NSAIDs.
- NSAIDs can cause acute and chronic papillary necrosis from medullary ischemic injury.
- The most common electrolyte abnormality seen with NSAIDs is hyponatremia.
- Other metabolic abnormalities include hyperkalemia and renal tubular acidosis type 4.
- NSAIDs cause fluid retention and worsen hypertension.

INTRODUCTION

Nonsteroidal antiinflammatory drugs (NSAIDs) have been around since 400 BC and used for their antipyretic, analgesic, and antiinflammatory properties. They were originally extracted from the bark and leaves of the willow tree; their use is recorded in the

---

Disclosures: none.
[a] Garden City Hospital, Michigan State University, 5001 Sheridan St, B44, Davenport, IA 52806, USA; [b] Nephrology Fellowship Program, St John Health System, Macomb-Oakland Campus, St. John Macomb Hospital, 12000 E. 12 Mile Road, Warren, MI 48093, USA; [c] Hypertension Nephrology Associate, PC, Livonia, MI, USA
* Corresponding author. Nephrology Fellowship Program, St John Health System, Macomb-Oakland Campus, Warren, MI.
E-mail address: Anthony875@comcast.net

Prim Care Clin Office Pract 41 (2014) 803–821
http://dx.doi.org/10.1016/j.pop.2014.09.001
0095-4543/14/$ – see front matter © 2014 Elsevier Inc. All rights reserved.

earliest civilizations, such as Sumer, Egypt, Assyria, and Greece. It was during late seventeenth century AD when the active ingredient of the willow extracts was identified as salicin in Europe. A German company by the name of Kolbe began mass production of salicylic acid; Bayer modified it and made it more palatable in 1899 as acetylsalicylic acid and marketed it as aspirin.[1] NSAIDs have evolved a great deal over the past century ever since Sir John Vane, an English pharmacologist, discovered the mechanism of action of NSAIDs, specifically their role in prostaglandin (PG) synthesis inhibition via the cyclooxygenase (COX) pathways.[2] With an increasing understanding of COX inhibition, NSAIDs have been used to manage a wide spectrum of medical problems, an exhaustive list ranging from minor aches, sprains, and fevers to chronic inflammatory conditions, such as rheumatic arthritis, osteoarthritis, inflammatory bowel disease, and crystal arthropathies like gout.[3] Over time, the excessive use of NSAIDs has made this class of drugs notorious for gastrointestinal bleeding, ulcers, platelet dysfunction syndrome, blood pressure dysregulation, and kidney disease.[4]

THE SCOPE OF THE PROBLEM

Inarguably NSAIDs are the most widely prescribed medications in the world today, with an estimate of more than 111 million prescriptions, and 30 billion over-the-counter doses administered annually in the United States to treat a multitude of conditions. It is estimated that 2.5 million Americans experience NSAID-mediated renal effects annually.[5,6] Risk factors that predispose patients to NSAID-induced renal functional alterations include age greater than 65 years; history of cardiovascular disease; diabetes; male sex; high NSAID dosage; concurrent use of other nephrotoxic drugs; and, most importantly, a history of chronic kidney disease (CKD) (estimated glomerular filtration rate [eGFR] <60 mL/min).[7] More than 20% of patients who take nonselective NSAIDs have more than one of these risk factors and may very well manifest alterations in renal function.[6] In a study published in 2011 with 12,000 patients greater than 20 years of age with CKD and NSAID use, 2.5% patients with mild CKD, 2.5% with moderate, and 5.0% with severe CKD were taking NSAIDS; 10% had prescriptions, whereas 66% had been taking it almost every day for more than a year.[8] It is, therefore, incumbent on the clinician to be cognizant of the side effects of NSAIDs in the light of renal function and exercise caution while prescribing treatment with both COX selective and nonselective NSAIDs. The reason for this is that, in addition to their role in inflammation, PGs are important regulators of vascular tone, salt and water balance, and renin release, which, when inhibited by COX inhibition, will cause adverse effects, including a multitude of acute and chronic complications.[9] This article highlights a few major complications, such as fluid retention and edema, hemodynamically mediated acute renal failure, acute interstitial nephritis, chronic analgesic nephropathy, electrolyte imbalances, nephrotic syndrome, and blood pressure dysregulation, which clinicians need to be aware of before administering NSAIDs for the management of pain and inflammation.

PROSTAGLANDINS, CYCLOOXYGENASE 1 AND 2, AND NONSTEROIDAL ANTIINFLAMMATORY DRUGS

The synthesis and physiology of PGs mediated by the two enzymes cyclooxygenase 1 and 2 (COX) begins with arachidonic acid (AA) (**Fig. 1**). AA is a 20 carbon unsaturated fatty acid embedded in the cellular membranes, which, on stimulation by an inflammatory process, is converted to PGs and thromboxanes. This process is mediated by enzymes called COX, lipoxygenase, and cytochrome P450.[10] Of significant note is that the committed step in the COX pathway is initiated by the two isoforms of COX,

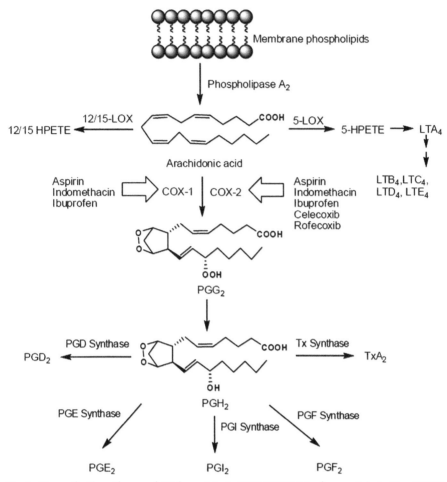

Fig. 1. Biosynthetic pathway of PG from AA via COX-1/COX-2 isoform catalysis. The NSAIDs aspirin, indomethacin, and ibuprofen are nonselective inhibitors of COX isozymes, whereas celecoxib and rofecoxib exhibit selective COX-2 inhibition. HPETE, hydroperoxyeicosatetraenoic acid; LOX, lipoxygenase. (*From* Rao PN. Evolution of nonsteroidal anti-inflammatory drugs (NSAIDs): cyclooxygenase (COX) inhibition and beyond. J Pharm Pharm Sci 2008;11(2):81s–110s.)

COX-1 and COX-2. AA is converted to PG G2, which is then converted to PG H2. PG H2, in turn, is converted to 5 biologically active PGs: PGD_2, PGE_2, PGF_{2a}, PGI_2, and thromboxane A_2.[11,12] The COX-1 isoform is involved in the regulation of normal physiologic processes and maintenance of the homeostatic state and, hence, is found in high levels in the cells and tissues, such as endothelium, monocytes, platelets, renal collecting tubules, gastrointestinal tract, and seminal vesicles.[13] This is evidenced by the fact that COX-1 enzyme does not seem to be affected by the inflammatory process because similar levels of mRNA and protein are detected in both normal and inflamed tissue in animal models.[14–16] The COX-2 enzyme is, however, induced by mediators of inflammation (lipopolysaccharide, interleukin-1, tumor necrosis factor, all in selective cells and tissues such as vascular endothelium, osteoclasts, and macrophages.[17–19] This phenomenon is evidenced by studies that have shown COX-2 to be nondetectable in normal tissue, but it is detectable after induction by inflammatory stimuli. Recent studies have demonstrated that COX-2 also plays specific functions in reproduction, renal physiology, bone resorption, and neurotransmission.[17–19] In conjunction with histamine and bradykinin, PGs, such as PGI_2, and PGE_2, promote inflammation via the COX-2 pathway, thus, worsening edema, vascular permeability, and pain. Hence, nonselective NSAIDs or COX-2 selective NSAIDs can downregulate the COX-2 pathway and inhibit the progression of inflammation.

Multiple assays have been used to study the selectivity of the available NSAIDs; by their selectivity to inhibit COX-1, versus COX-2 or both, NSAIDS have been classified in 4 major categories (**Table 1**).[20]

CYCLOOXYGENASE AND THE KIDNEYS

Contrary to the functions of COX-1 and COX-2 as described earlier, the kidneys are interesting in the way that both COX-1 and COX-2 simultaneously participate in the normal physiology of the renal function.[21] COX-1 is expressed constitutively in the kidney and has been localized to collecting ducts, arteriolar endothelial cells, mesangial cells, and epithelial cells of the Bowman capsule; COX-2 is expressed in the macula densa, epithelial cells lining the ascending loop of Henle, and the medullary interstitial cells of the renal papillae.[12] Overall both COX-1 and COX-2 are involved in regulating the GFR, sodium regulation, blood pressure regulation in conjunction with the renin-angiotensin-aldosterone pathway, and volume regulation. COX-2 is also involved in renal development as evidenced by reports of renal dysgenesis and oligohydramnios in the offspring of women who took nonselective NSAIDs during the third trimester of pregnancy. PGs and their inhibition by COX-2 and nonselective COX inhibitors have been implicated in the process of normal renal development (**Box 1**).[22,23]

ACUTE KIDNEY INJURY
Hemodynamically Mediated Injury

Recent studies have shown that hemodynamically mediated acute kidney injury (AKI) can occur from both nonspecific NSAIDs and selective COX-2 enzyme inhibitor

Table 1
Classification of NSAIDs according to their COX-1/2 inhibitory activities. Please notice that Rofecoxib (Vioxx) has not been included in Table 1 as it has been removed from the market by the FDA because of its severe cardiovascular side effects

Class	Properties	Examples
Group 1	NSAIDs that inhibit both COX-1 and COX-2 completely with little selectivity	Aspirin, ibuprofen, diclofenac, indomethacin, naproxen, piroxicam
Group 2	NSAIDs that inhibit COX-2 with a 5- to 50-fold selectivity	Celecoxib, etodolac, meloxicam, nimesulide
Group 3	NSAIDs that inhibit COX-2 with a >50-fold selectivity	Rofecoxib, NS-398
Group 4	NSAIDs that are weak inhibitors of both isoforms	5-Aminosalicylic acid, sodium salicylate, nabumetone, sulfasalazine

From Rao PN, et al. Evolution of nonsteroidal anti-inflammatory drugs (NSAIDs): cyclooxygenase (COX) inhibition and beyond. J Pharm Pharm Sci 2008;11(2):81s–110s.

Box 1
NSAIDs, COX inhibition, and dysregulation of renal function

COX inhibition–induced renal

Acute kidney injury: hemodynamically mediated ischemic injury

Acute kidney injury: acute (tubulonephritis) interstitial nephritis

Acute kidney injury: glomerulonephropathy (minimal change disease)

Papillary necrosis

Electrolyte abnormalities: hyperkalemia

Electrolyte abnormalities: hyponatremia

Electrolyte abnormalities: renal tubular acidosis

CKD

Dysregulation of blood pressure control and other cardiovascular diseases

Edema

NSAIDs.[24–30] According to one study, up to 15% cases of AKI are caused by NSAIDs; in patients older than 65 years, the rate can be greater than 25%.[31] Renal PGs cause vasodilatation of afferent vessels and assist in maintaining normal GFR. This function of PGs is further amplified in the setting of an acute ischemic or hypotensive event whereby other mediators come into play, such as angiotensin II, norepinephrine, endothelin, and vasopressin, where PGs cause afferent vasodilatation to maintain adequate perfusion and minimize ischemia. In the event of COX inhibition via selective and nonselective NSAIDs, this ability of maintaining adequate GFR is compromised, thus resulting in a drop in the renal hydraulic pressure in the peritubular capillaries, thereby causing ischemic injury and increasing the risk of acute tubular necrosis (ATN).[26,29] PGs are also synthesized by macula densa cells and maintain a check on those cells' synthesis of renin, which becomes accentuated under COX inhibition, which would result in amplification of the renin-angiotensin-aldosterone pathway that causes sodium reabsorption, edema, and worsening of hypertension. A review of recent data shows that the pathologic phenomenon described earlier get accentuated when NSAIDs are taken in the setting of heart failure, administration of radioactive contrast, angiotensin-converting enzyme inhibitor (ACEI), angiotensin receptor blockers (ARBs), and intravascular volume depletion[30,32,33] as the combination impairs renal blood flow autoregulation. The reason for this observation is that under the normal circumstances, PGs are synthesized at low basal levels and their function is also not very significant. However, under the conditions whereby the body is in a state of decreased effective arterial circulation, such as cirrhosis, heart failure, or in a state of decreased intravascular volume, CKD and chronic hypercalcemia kidneys will increase the generation of PGs that will maintain patency of renal arteries by vasodilatation to maintain a steady-state GFR. **Fig. 2** shows a schematic of the phenomenon described earlier.

Clinical Presentation

In the clinical setting, patients will have an elevated serum creatinine and little to no proteinuria (<500 mg). Lack of proteinuria and hematuria with a positive presence of granular and epithelial cell casts is the classic description of ischemic injury, especially that seen after 3 to 7 days of taking NSAIDs. The presence of leukocytes is classically

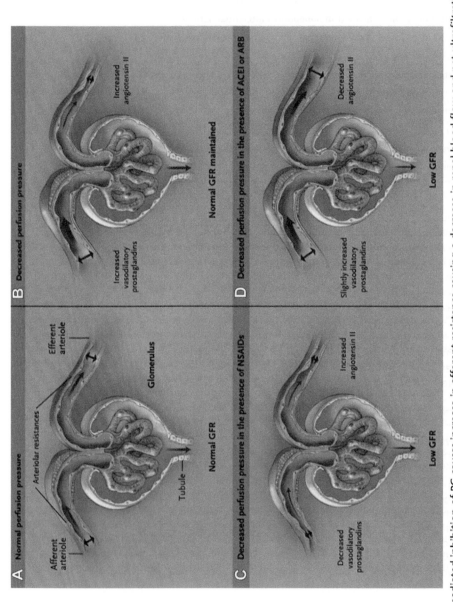

Fig. 2. NSAID-mediated inhibition of PG causes increase in afferent resistance causing a decrease in renal blood flow and net ultrafiltration pressure. (*From* Abuelo J. Normotensive ischemic acute renal failure. N Engl J Med 2007;357:797–805.)

not seen in ATN, but their presence should have the clinician consider the possibility of acute interstitial nephritis (AIN) caused by NSAIDs. New-onset proteinuria, especially greater than 1 g in 24 hours, should warrant a work-up of glomerulonephritis, especially minimal change disease, which is also a complication of NSAIDs use.

Management

The treatment of NSAID-induced AKI is immediate cessation of NSAIDs and volume resuscitation if volume depletion is an issue. The overall management of AKI other than immediate cessation of the drug is not very different from the overall care of AKI from other causes as guided by the clinical presentation and work-up that follows.

Guidelines for Managing Patients with Acute Kidney Injury

1. It is important for the clinicians to be aware of the groups of people who are at an increased risk of NSAID-induced hemodynamically mediated AKI. The following is a list of patients in whom care should be taken before prescribing nonspecific as well as COX-2–specific NSAIDs[34]:
   - CKD, eGFR less than 60 mL/min per 1.73 m^2
   - Intravascular volume depletion (eg, from aggressive diuresis, vomiting, diarrhea, pancreatitis, burns)
   - Effective arterial volume depletion (eg, heart failure, nephrotic syndrome, or cirrhosis)
   - Older age, especially older than 60 years
   - Hypercalcemia
   - Renal artery stenosis
   - Medications, such as ACEIs, ARBs, calcineurin inhibitors, aminoglycoside antibiotics
   - Intravascular administration of radiocontrast dye
2. In the abovementioned high-risk patients, NSAIDs, both nonspecific as well as COX-2 specific, should be kept at a minimum, especially for chronic use. However, in patients with a GFR 60 to 90 mL/min, for an acute illness, debility, and flare of a chronic inflammation such as gout, clinicians should attempt to volume resuscitate first, then administer NSAIDs with caution and closely monitor creatinine and urine.
3. For patients in the high-risk group, who have an acute inflammatory condition and have a GFR less than 60 mL/min, medications other than NSAIDs ought to be considered for management of pain and inflammation, such as a short course of steroids: oral/intravenous/intramuscular/intra-articular/topical preparations depending on the case, opioid analgesics, acetaminophen, for palliation. For more specific cases, such as gouty attacks, colchicine may be used instead of NSAIDs with dose adjustment for renal function.
4. Definitely avoid giving NSAIDs before getting intravenous radiocontrast.
5. If conservative management including adequate volume resuscitation and cessation of NSAIDs does not improve renal function in 7 days, then other causes of AKI must be considered and the possibility of renal biopsy should be given a thought.

ACUTE INTERSTITIAL NEPHRITIS

AIN accounts for approximately 15% of cases of AKI. It is a condition characterized by worsening of renal function caused by an acute inflammation and edema of the renal interstitium often accompanied by tubulitis by infiltration of lymphocytes and eosinophils (**Fig. 3**). There are several causes of this condition; but medications account for

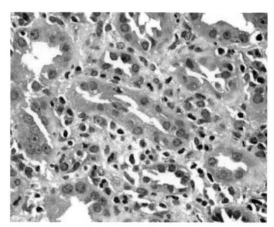

Fig. 3. Drug-induced AIN with prominent interstitial inflammation characterized by lymphocytes, eosinophils, and focal plasma cells. Renal biopsy sample (hematoxylin-eosin, original magnification ×600). (*From* Perazella MA, Markowitz GS. Drug-induced acute interstitial nephritis. Nat Rev Nephrol 2010;6:461–70; with permission.)

nearly 75% of the cases studied, of which NSAIDs are by far the most common cause.[35] Other less common conditions that cause AIN are infections, followed by inflammatory conditions, such as systemic lupus erythematosus. Both COX-2–specific and nonspecific NSAIDs are equally incriminated among the medications that can cause AIN.[36]

Clinical Presentation

Clinically patients may present with a myriad of symptoms, mostly nonspecific, such as nausea, anorexia, and malaise, which are frequently associated with AKI; some patients may even present with oliguria. The classically described features of AIN (ie, fever, rash, and eosinophilia) are not as common as they were thought to be, according to the most recent data, especially when it was presumed that AIN was caused by NSAIDs.[37] In several studies and case series, fever and rashes accounted for less than 15%; the triad of fever, rash, and eosinophilia was present in less than 10% of the cases of AIN.[38] More recently, eosinophiluria, defined as eosinophils greater than 5% of urinary leukocytes or greater than 1% of urinary leukocytes by Hansel stain, is under investigation to evaluate its efficacy to rule in AIN. Unfortunately, most studies have shown variability in sensitivity and specificity of eosinophiluria for AIN; but overall this test is at best 70% to 90% specific and sensitive for AIN.[39] Lack of it does not exclude the condition. It is important to note that eosinophiluria becomes very helpful when seen concomitantly with a biopsy showing acute inflammatory changes. Another feature that may assist the clinician in making the diagnosis is the analysis of urine sediment that may show leukocytes and also occasionally leukocyte casts. Urinalysis may also show proteinuria of less than 0.5 g/24 h, although it is rare.[39]

Management

Once the clinician has made the diagnosis of AIN, the next step is its appropriate management. The most important principle of managing AIN is prompt cessation of the drug that is thought to have caused the disease.[39] The typical prognosis is that patients will improve within 1 week, and serum creatinine may return back to baseline but not always. In some cases, patients may even progress to have CKD from chronic interstitial nephritis. Studies have shown that some patients may also end up on dialysis, but eventually only less than 10% of patients remain dialysis dependent in the long run.[40] Patients who developed AIN with a short course of NSAIDs are more likely to improve renal function than those who took greater than 3 weeks of medication. Patients who do not improve after prompt cessation of the offending agent have been challenging, and various investigators have tried several options with variable results. Before initiating any medications, it is important to obtain a biopsy to confirm the diagnosis. Several studies have evaluated steroids for treating patients with AIN. Once AIN is established, based on several trials, a possible regimen is prednisone 0.5 to 1.0 mg/kg/d up to 60 mg/d for 4 weeks, then taper off when renal function returns to near baseline.[41] Studies have shown variable results with glucocorticoids. Some have shown improvement of GFR faster than the control group, whereas other studies showed no difference compared with the control arm when the treatment was cessation of the offending drug. Some patients have shown resistance to glucocorticoid therapy; unfortunately, patients with NSAID-induced AIN have frequently been steroid-resistant patients who did not initially improve with cessation of the offending drug.[42] Some small case studies and anecdotal studies have used mycophenolate mofetil, cyclophosphamide, and cyclosporine with variable results.[43,44] It is important for the clinician to bear in mind that if proteinuria is more than 1 g/24 h, then a concomitant T-cell–mediated podocyte injury (ie, a glomerulonephropathy, more specifically minimal change disease [MCD]) secondary to NSAIDs should be considered.[45] This syndrome (ie, AIN with MCD) is a self-limited disease; hence, treatment is limited to withdrawal of the offending agent. In some cases, a short course of steroids has shown benefit. Renal function typically returns to normal in 1 month to 1 year.[46]

Minimal Change Disease

Several investigators have reported secondary MCD from NSAIDs without the interstitial inflammation; however, MCD with interstitial nephritis is the more commonly seen variant.[47] Exactly how NSAIDs cause MCD is yet to be understood. A proposed mechanism is that NSAID-mediated COX inhibition causes preferential conversion of arachidonic acid to leukotriene, which in turn causes activation of helper T lymphocytes that infiltrate the glomeruli and cause podocyte injury.[34,46,48] Both selective and nonselective COX-2 NSAIDs can cause this pattern of injury.[34,46,48,49] One study looking at minimal change glomerulopathy associated with NSAIDs concluded that up to 10% of the cases of MCD may be attributable to NSAIDs,[50] of whose treatment initially is cessation of the offending agent, followed by glucocorticoids if cessation of the drug does not reverse the injury. Some studies have shown a benefit of using corticosteroids. In extreme conditions whereby patients are resistant to corticosteroids, then other agents, such as cyclophosphamide and cyclosporine, have shown variable results to achieve remission.[51]

PAPILLARY NECROSIS

NSAIDs have been reported to cause acute, subacute, and chronic papillary necrosis, which forms the basis of analgesic nephropathy.[52–54] Analgesic nephropathy rates have considerably declined since the 1990s when phenacetin was taken off the market, which was infamous for causing analgesic nephropathy, as evidenced by literature from Europe, United States, and Australia.[55] Papillary necrosis becomes a serious concern in the conditions of depleted intravascular volume,[56] such as vomiting, diarrhea, sepsis, lack of oral intake, and use of medications such as diuretics while taking NSAIDs. The renal medullary and papillary regions are further downstream to the rich blood supply in the cortical areas; hence, those regions depend on PG-mediated vasodilatation to maintain adequate perfusion and oxygenation. In the event of a COX-2 or a nonspecific NSAID-mediated inhibition of this phenomenon, the papillary and medullary regions become ischemic and eventually necrotic, thereby causing renal failure. Because COX-2 is found in the cells of the medullary area of the kidney, it becomes very important for the survival of the cells in a hypertonic medium. This setting raises the concern of an increasing risk of papillary necrosis in the long-term use of COX-2–selective NSAIDs.

Clinical Presentation

People who develop papillary necrosis after chronic NSAID use are typically older than 45 years and typically do not complain of any symptoms.[57] Some patients, up to 60%, especially women, may have recurrent urinary tract infections. Hypertension is another common finding in more than 70% of patients. The diagnosis should be considered when the serum creatinine is found to be elevated and urinalysis is positive for sterile pyuria. Imaging, especially computed tomography (CT) scan, is another effective way to make the diagnosis (**Fig. 4**). Frequently imaging does not demonstrate anatomic injury consistent with this entity, in which case the clinician should also consider other diagnoses, such as medullary sponge kidney disease, myeloma kidney, sarcoidosis, and infections, such as tuberculosis. The overall prognosis of renal function is a function of time: the time the disease was diagnosed and when the medication was discontinued. Studies have shown that renal function will continue to deteriorate if medications continue to be administered. A study published in 2003 showed a 6-fold increased risk of reaching the combined end point of death or dialysis in patients who continued to use analgesics, including NSAIDs.[58] Multiple studies over the past decades have shown that aspirin is generally not nephrotoxic, especially if taken in low doses; but in this condition, even aspirin has been shown to worsen renal function. It is important to remember that other entities can cause papillary necrosis, such as diabetic nephropathy, sickle cell nephropathy, urinary tract obstruction, and renal tuberculosis.

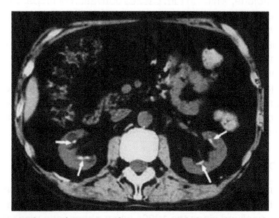

Fig. 4. Non–contrast-enhanced CT scan of a patient with long-time analgesic abuse showed thinning of the renal parenchyma and typical papillary calcifications (*arrows*). (*From* Floege J, Johnson RJ, Feehall J. Comprehensive clinical nephrology. 4th edition. Philadelphia: Elsevier; 2011; with permission. *Courtesy of* Dr. Yoshifumi Ubara, Toranomon Hospital, Tokyo, Japan.)

NONSTEROIDAL ANTIINFLAMMATORY DRUGS AND ELECTROLYTE IMBALANCES
Hyponatremia

PGs play an important role in the regulation of vasopressin (ADH). When an NSAID is administered, it blocks the PG's effects on ADH's function of free-water clearance. As a result of this, the nephron tends to absorb free water and thereby causes hyponatremia.[59] NSAIDs have also shown to exacerbate thiazide diuretic–mediated hyponatremia in the elderly population.[60] While on the subject of sodium imbalances caused by NSAIDs, it is important to highlight the fact that NSAIDs remove the inhibitory effect of PGs on sodium reabsorption, which leads to sodium retention and edema.[61] With prolonged therapy, even healthy individuals with no major cardiovascular diseases may have a weight gain of as much as 0.5 to 1.0 kg, whereas the degree of sodium and water retention may be more prominent in patients with underlying heart failure or cirrhosis. Another problem caused by this phenomenon is relative resistance to diuretics associated with NSAID therapy, which may worsen and exacerbate heart failure.

Hyperkalemia

NSAIDs can cause hyperkalemia by 2 distinct mechanisms. First, they can inhibit the PG-mediated secretion of renin and downregulate the renin-angiotensin-aldosterone pathway, thus, causing decreased potassium secretion in the principal cells of the collecting duct, resulting in hyperkalemia.[62,63] The second mechanism is by causing acute renal failure, which in turn decreases the GFR. This reduction in GFR decreases sodium delivery to the distal nephron and results in decreased secretion of potassium via the sodium-potassium exchanger. These two phenomena are much more pronounced in patients who have intravascular volume depletion, heart failure, or who are on medications such as ACEI, ARB and Aldosterone blockers.

Renal Tubular Acidosis

As mentioned earlier, NSAIDs can cause hyporeninemic hypoaldosteronism, which causes hyperkalemia. Prolonged hyperkalemia causes dysregulation of ammoniogenesis and also decreases net renal acid excretion in the form of ammonium ions in the distal nephron and causes renal tubular acidosis type 4, a type of hyperchloremic metabolic acidosis. In this entity, the kidney's ability to acidify the urine in an acid load is relatively intact and urine pH is usually less than 5.5.[64] In a study of 50 hospitalized patients that were given indomethacin, about 34% developed hyperkalemia by 0.5 to 0.9 meq/L, and about 26% developed hyperkalemia with an increase in serum potassium by 1 meq/L.[65] An important point worth mentioning here is that renal tubular acidosis (RTA) type 4 is typically seen in patients with CKD, such as diabetic nephropathy or chronic interstitial nephritis; but it may be seen purely from medications, such as NSAIDS and calcineurin inhibitors, in which case the hyperkalemia and RTA resolves completely once the offending medication has been discontinued.[66]

Role of Cyclooxygenase 2 Selective and Nonselective Nonsteroidal Antiinflammatory Drugs in Hypertension

Multiple studies have shown that both COX-1 and COX-2 inhibitors block PG-mediated natriuresis and vasodilatation, thereby causing sodium retention by more than 30%, fluid retention, vasoconstriction that eventually leads to edema, and elevated blood pressure.[67] Under normal circumstances, a healthy kidney will mount a response to this physiologic derangement and will upregulate natriuresis to maintain the steady-state homeostasis; thus, the clinical side effects may not be so severe. However, patients who have CKD and are unable to regulate the excess sodium; fluid load will also eventually develop worsening of edema, hypertension, and eventually heart failure. These side effects may manifest as early as 1 to 2 weeks of initiating therapy with NSAIDs.[67]

More recently, another cause for worsening of hypertension has been studied (ie, effects of NSAIDs on aldosterone metabolism). Several nonselective NSAIDs block the glucuronidation of aldosterone by human kidney microsomes that increase plasma and tissue concentrations of aldosterone.[68] Increasing levels of circulating aldosterone will cause sodium retention and endothelial injury, myocardial fibrosis, and left ventricular remodeling, all of which will precipitate worsening of hypertension, edema, and heart failure. Contemporary clinical research is investigating NSAIDs and their destabilization of blood pressure in hypertensive patients being treated with antihypertensive medications, including ACEI or ARBs, beta-blockers, calcium channel blockers, or diuretics.[67] A recently published trial studied the effects of celecoxib and diclofenac on ambulatory blood pressure and GFRs in a double-blind crossover study. The mean 24-hour systolic blood pressure was significantly increased by diclofenac (mean 4.2 mm Hg) compared with celecoxib (mean 0.6 mm Hg), and GFR was significantly reduced by diclofenac but not by celecoxib. The investigators thought that these differences were attributable in part to the once-daily dosing of celecoxib versus the twice-daily dosing of diclofenac.[69]

A larger trial using the clinic systolic blood pressure as the primary end point evaluated the effects of rofecoxib 25 mg/d and celecoxib 200 mg/d in 1092 patients on chronic, stable doses of antihypertensive therapies. This study showed that rofecoxib induced significant increases in systolic blood pressure in patients who were taking ACEIs and beta-blockers but not in those who were taking calcium channel blockers (**Fig. 5**). These results support the notion that calcium antagonists do not significantly depend on vascular prostacyclin as part of their mechanism of action. Alternatively,

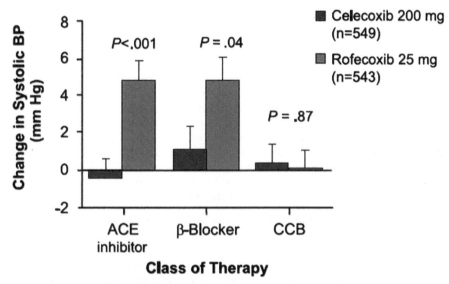

Fig. 5. Effects of rofecoxib and celecoxib on clinic systolic blood pressure (BP) in patients given ACEIs, beta-blockers, and calcium antagonists. Destabilization occurred after 6 weeks of treatment with rofecoxib in patients taking ACEIs and beta-blockers but not in those taking calcium antagonists. Celecoxib did not affect systolic BP control rates in the antihypertensive drug treatment groups. (*From* White WB, et al. Cardiovascular effects of the cyclooxygenase inhibitors. Hypertension 2007;49:408–18; with permission.)

calcium antagonists may not be influenced by increases in total body sodium as are the ACEI, diuretics, and blockers of the sympathetic nervous system.[70] In another trial comparing 2 nonspecific NSAIDs, neither ibuprofen nor naproxen significantly increased mean blood pressure in patients treated with chronic verapamil therapy.[71] Another study also showed this finding with patients on nicardipine who were treated with naproxen.[72]

The Celecoxib Rofecoxib Efficacy and Safety in Comorbidities Evaluation Trial was a comprehensive randomized, double-blind clinical trial evaluating the effects of NSAIDs in treated hypertensive subjects on ACEIs alone or in combination with other classes of antihypertensive therapy. The primary end point was change from baseline in the 24-hour ambulatory systolic blood pressure after 6 and 12 weeks of therapy with celecoxib, naproxen, or rofecoxib in 400 patients with type 2 diabetes, hypertension, and osteoarthritis. This study demonstrated that, at equally effective doses for osteoarthritis, treatment with rofecoxib 25 mg daily induced a significant destabilization of 24-hour systolic blood pressure control compared with celecoxib 200 mg daily and naproxen 500 mg twice daily. Thirty percent of patients administered rofecoxib had a resultant 24-hour systolic blood pressure of greater than 135 mm Hg compared with 16% of patients randomly assigned to celecoxib and 19% to naproxen. Baseline clinical characteristics of the patients enrolled in the study did not predict worsening of hypertension caused by COX-2 or nonselective NSAIDs. During the course of the study, significantly more patients developed peripheral edema while taking rofecoxib compared with the other 2 treatment groups, but no patient developed kidney dysfunction (**Fig. 6**).[73]

Coadministration of NSAIDs or COX-2 selective inhibitors with antihypertensive agents is quite common.[67] Meta-analyses of the NSAIDs from the early 1990s showed that NSAIDs could increase mean arterial pressure by as much as 5 to 6 mm Hg in hypertensive patients.[74] This magnitude of elevation in blood pressure caused by NSAIDs is significant as demonstrated by clinical trials. Hypertension especially a concern in the elderly population as it is associated with increases in the risk of both ischemic and hemorrhagic stroke, congestive heart failure, and ischemic cardiac events.[67] In the VALUE study, differences of 4 mm Hg in systolic blood pressure control in an older population of hypertensive patients randomly assigned to 2 treatment groups (valsartan and amlodipine) resulted in a clinically and statistically significant relative increase in cardiac events of 40% in the less well-controlled group (valsartan recipients) during the first 6 months of the trial.[75] NSAIDs and COX-2 inhibitors should be used with caution in hypertensive patients who are taking ACEIs, ARBs, or beta-blockers as well as in patients who have diabetes or mild kidney disease. Patients with congestive heart failure are particularly at an increased for developing exacerbations of heart failure and increased hospitalizations as seen in the study arm with NSAIDs and COX-2 inhibitors, comparing them with non-NSAIDs users in one of the largest trials published in California.[76] If a clinician chooses to use NSAIDs for an acute treatment of an inflammatory process, such as gout or migraine, for patients with a history of heart failure, left ventricular hypertrophy, or hypertension, it is recommended to follow those patients carefully in short intervals, in 1 to 3 weeks of initiation of therapy, and assess their renal function, blood pressure, and assessment of their cardiovascular condition (**Fig. 7**, **Table 2**).

A FINAL WORD ON CHRONIC KIDNEY DISEASE

Clinicians should exercise caution while administering NSAIDs to patients who have chronically reduced GFR less than 60 mL/min. NSAIDs, both COX-2 and nonselective,

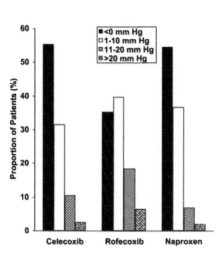

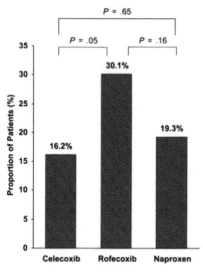

Normotensive: Ambulatory Systolic Blood Pressure <135 mm Hg
Hypertensive: Ambulatory Systolic Blood Pressure ≥ 135 mm Hg

Fig. 6. Effects of celecoxib, rofecoxib, and naproxen on changes in 24-hour mean systolic blood pressure (*left*) and on proportion of patients who destabilized to hypertensive values (*right*) after 6 weeks of therapy. ABPM, ambulatory systolic blood pressure. (*From* White WB, et al. Cardiovascular effects of the cyclooxygenase inhibitors. Hypertension 2007;49:408–18; with permission.)

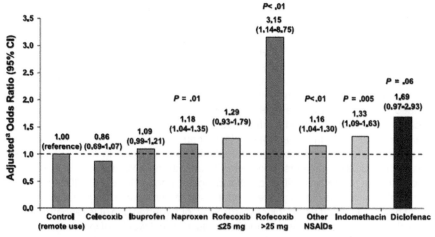

[a]Adjusted for age, gender, health plan region, medical history, smoking, and medication use.

Fig. 7. Results of a 2-year observational study in 1.4 million persons administered various NSAIDs in a closed, formulary health maintenance organization in California. The relative risk of acute myocardial infarction and sudden cardiovascular death was compared with nonusers of NSAIDs and COX-2 inhibitors (control group). CI, confidence interval. (*From* White WB, et al. Cardiovascular effects of the cyclooxygenase inhibitors. Hypertension 2007;49:408–18; with permission.)

Table 2
Summary of observation findings on the cardiovascular risk of inhibitors of COX

Drug	Relative Risk of Event	95% CI
Celecoxib	1.06	0.91–1.23
Diclofenac	1.40	1.16–1.70
Ibuprofen	1.07	0.97–1.18
Indomethacin	1.30	1.07–1.60
Meloxicam	1.25	1.00–1.55
Naproxen	0.97	0.81–1.07
Rofecoxib (<25 mg)	1.33	1.00–1.70
Rofecoxib (>25 mg)	2.19	1.69–2.91

Abbreviation: CI, confidence interval.
From White WB, et al. Cardiovascular effects of the cyclooxygenase inhibitors. Hypertension 2007;49:408–18; with permission.

cause inhibition of PG-mediated vasodilatation, thereby causing decreased renal perfusion and further worsening of GFR. Because low doses of NSAIDs can precipitate renal failure, there is really no safe dose of NSAIDs in patients with CKD. Patients with CKD are also susceptible to developing worsening of CKD because of papillary necrosis from NSAIDs. Another reason to keep patients with CKD off of NSAIDs is to decrease their risk of developing AKI, as each assault further causes their CKD to worsen over time. Patients who have CKD are often on treatment with ACEIs and ARBs and diuretics for blood pressure, proteinuria, and volume control. These medications interact with NSAIDs and may worsen their blood pressure control, cause fluid retention, and increase the risk of developing cardiovascular disease. Elderly patients and patients with CKD need to be asked if they are taking any NSAIDs routinely, and they should be counseled on the adverse effects of NSAIDs. It is very tempting for patients to take NSAIDs, as they are effective analgesics and antiinflammatory medicines. Unfortunately, it is quite often the elderly population that deals with issues of chronic pain, osteoarthritis, gout, and chronic inflammation.

REFERENCES

1. Vane JR. The fight against rheumatism: from willow bark to COX-1 sparing drugs. J Physiol Pharmacol 2000;51:573–86.
2. Vane JR. Inhibition of prostaglandin synthesis as a mechanism of action for aspirin-like drugs. Nat New Biol 1971;43:232–5.
3. Vane JR. The mode of action of aspirin and similar compounds. J Allergy Clin Immunol 1976;58:691–712.
4. Moncada S, Ferreira SH, Vane JR. Prostaglandins, aspirin-like drugs and the oedema of inflammation. Nature 1973;246:217–9.
5. Singh G, Triadafilopoulos G. Epidemiology of NSAID induced gastrointestinal complications. J Rheumatol 1999;26(Suppl 56):18–24.
6. Harris RC, Breyer MD. Update on cyclo-oxygenase inhibitors. Clin J Am Soc Nephrol 2006;1:236–45.
7. Johnson AG. NSAIDs and increased blood pressure. What is the clinical significance? Drug Saf 1997;17:277–89.
8. Plantinga L, Grubbs V, Sarkar U, et al. Nonsteroidal anti-inflammatory drug use among persons with chronic kidney disease in the United States. Ann Fam Med 2011;9:423–30.

9. Sandhu GK, Heyneman CA. Nephrotoxic potential of selective cyclooxygenase-2 inhibitors. Ann Pharmacother 2004;38:700–4.

10. Smith W, DeWitt DL, Garavito RM. Cyclooxygenases: structural, cellular, and molecular biology. Annu Rev Biochem 2000;69:145–82.

11. Abramovitz M. Prostanoid receptors. Annu Rep Med Chem 1998;33:223–31.

12. FitzGerald GA, Patrono C. The coxibs, selective inhibitors of cyclooxygenase-2. N Engl J Med 2001;345:433–42.

13. Smith WL. Prostaglandin endoperoxide H synthases-1 and -2. Adv Immunol 1996;62:167–215.

14. Smith CJ, Yan Zhang, Koboldt CM, et al. Pharmacological analysis of cyclooxygenase-1 in inflammation. Proc Natl Acad Sci U S A 1998;95:13313–8.

15. Lee SH, Soyoola E, Chanmugam P, et al. Selective expression of mitogen inducible cyclooxygenase in macrophages stimulated with lipopolysaccharide. J Biol Chem 1992;267:25943–8.

16. Seibert K, Zhang Y, Leahy K, et al. Pharmacological and biochemical demonstration of the role of cyclooxygenase-2 in inflammation and pain. Proc Natl Acad Sci U S A 1994;91:12013–7.

17. Lim H. Multiple female reproductive failures in cyclooxygenase-2 deficient mice. Cell 1997;91:197–208.

18. Cheng HF, Wang J-L, Zhang M-Z, et al. Angiotensin II attenuates renal cortical cyclooxygenase-2 expression. J Clin Invest 1999;103:953–61.

19. Breder CD. Characterization of inducible cyclooxygenase in rat brain. J Comp Neurol 1995;355:296–315.

20. Rao PN, Knaus EE. Evolution of nonsteroidal anti-inflammatory drugs (NSAIDs): cyclooxygenase (COX) inhibition and beyond. J Pharm Pharm Sci 2008;11(2):81s–110s.

21. Vane JR, Bakhle YS, Botting RM. Cyclooxygenases 1 and 2. Annu Rev Pharmacol Toxicol 1998;38:97–120.

22. Voyer LE, Drut R, Méndez JH. Fetal renal maldevelopment with oligohydramnios following maternal use of piroxicam. Pediatr Nephrol 1994;8:592–4.

23. Veersema D, de Jong PA, van Wijck JA. Indomethacin and the fetal renal nonfunction syndrome. Eur J Obstet Gynecol Reprod Biol 1983;16:113–21.

24. Haragsim L, Dalal R, Bagga H, et al. Ketorolac-induced acute renal failure and hyperkalemia: report of three cases. Am J Kidney Dis 1994;24(4):578.

25. Oates JA, FitzGerald GA, Branch RA, et al. Clinical implications of prostaglandin and thromboxane A2 formation. N Engl J Med 1988;319(11):689–98.

26. Patrono C, Dunn MJ. The clinical significance of inhibition of renal prostaglandin synthesis. Kidney Int 1987;32(1):1.

27. Perazella MA. COX-2 selective inhibitors: analysis of the renal effects. Expert Opin Drug Saf 2002;1(1):53–64.

28. Perazella MA, Tray K. Selective cyclooxygenase-2 inhibitors: a pattern of nephrotoxicity similar to traditional nonsteroidal anti-inflammatory drugs. Am J Med 2001;111(1):64.

29. Schneider V, Levesque LE, Zhang B, et al. Association of selective and conventional nonsteroidal antiinflammatory drugs with acute renal failure: a population-based, nested case-control analysis. Am J Epidemiol 2006;164(9):881.

30. Huerta C, Castellsague J, Varas-Lorenzo C, et al. Nonsteroidal anti-inflammatory drugs and risk of ARF in the general population. Am J Kidney Dis 2005;45(3):531.

31. Kleinknecht D, Landais P, Goldfarb B. Pathophysiology and clinical aspects of drug-induced tubular necrosis in man. Contrib Nephrol 1987;55:145–58.

32. Lapi F, Azoulay L, Yin H, et al. Concurrent use of diuretics, angiotensin converting enzyme inhibitors, and angiotensin receptor blockers with non-steroidal anti-inflammatory drugs and risk of acute kidney injury: nested case-control study. BMJ 2013;346:e8525.
33. Heyman SN, Brezis M, Epstein FH, et al. Early renal medullary hypoxic injury from radiocontrast and indomethacin. Kidney Int 1991;40(4):632–42.
34. Clive DM, Stoff JS. Renal syndromes associated with nonsteroidal antiinflammatory drugs. N Engl J Med 1984;310(9):563–72.
35. Schwarz A. The outcome of acute interstitial nephritis: risk factors for the transition from acute to chronic interstitial nephritis. Clin Nephrol 2000; 54(3):179.
36. Esteve JB. COX-2 inhibitors and acute interstitial nephritis: case report and review of the literature. Clin Nephrol 2005;63(5):385.
37. Rossert J. Drug-induced acute interstitial nephritis. Kidney Int 2001;60:804–17.
38. Praga M. Acute interstitial nephritis. Kidney Int 2010;77(11):956.
39. Perazella NA, Markowitz GS. Drug-induced acute interstitial nephritis. Nat Rev Nephrol 2010;6:461–70.
40. Baker RJ, Pusey CD. The changing profile of acute tubulointerstitial nephritis. Nephrol Dial Transplant 2004;19:8–11.
41. Gonzales E, Gutiérrez E, Galeano C, et al. Early steroid treatment improves the recovery of renal function in patients with drug-induced acute interstitial nephritis. Kidney Int 2008;73(8):940.
42. Clarkson MR, Giblin L, O'Connell FP, et al. Acute interstitial nephritis: clinical features and response to corticosteroid therapy. Nephrol Dial Transplant 2004; 19(11):2778.
43. Preddle DC, Markowitz GS, Radhakrishnan J, et al. Mycophenolate mofetil for the treatment of interstitial nephritis. Clin J Am Soc Nephrol 2006;1(4):718.
44. Zuliani E. Vancomycin-induced hypersensitivity reaction with acute renal failure: resolution following cyclosporine treatment. Clin Nephrol 2005;64(2):155.
45. Gaughan WJ, Sheth VR, Francos GC, et al. Ranitidine-induced acute interstitial nephritis with epithelial cell foot process fusion. Am J Kidney Dis 1993;22(2): 337.
46. Levin ML. Patterns of tubulo-interstitial damage associated with nonsteroidal antiinflammatory drugs. Semin Nephrol 1988;8:55–61.
47. Kleinknecht D. Interstitial nephritis, the nephrotic syndrome, and chronic renal failure secondary to nonsteroidal anti-inflammatory drugs. Semin Nephrol 1995;15:228–35.
48. Abraham PA, Keane WF. Glomerular and interstitial disease induced by nonsteroidal anti- inflammatory drugs. Am J Nephrol 1984;4:1–6.
49. Alper AB Jr, Meleg-Smith S, Krane NK. Nephrotic syndrome and interstitial nephritis associated with celecoxib. Am J Kidney Dis 2002;40:1086–90.
50. Warren GV, Korbet SM, Schwartz MM, et al. Minimal change glomerulopathy associated with nonsteroidal antiinflammatory drugs. Am J Kidney Dis 1989; 13(2):127.
51. Matsumoto H, Nakao T, Okada T, et al. Initial remission-inducing effect of very low-dose cyclosporin monotherapy for minimal-change nephrotic syndrome in Japanese adults. Clin Nephrol 2001;55(2):143.
52. Atta MG, Whelton A. Acute renal papillary necrosis induced by ibuprofen. Am J Ther 1997;4:55–60.
53. DeBroe M, Elseviers M. Analgesic nephropathy. N Engl J Med 1998;338: 446–52.

54. Segasothy M, Samad S, Zulfigar A, et al. Chronic renal disease and papillary necrosis associated with the long-term use of nonsteroidal anti-inflammatory drugs as the sole or predominant analgesic. Am J Kidney Dis 1994;24: 17–24.

55. Mihatsch MJ, Khanlari B, Brunner FP. Obituary to analgesic nephropathy—an autopsy study. Nephrol Dial Transplant 2006;21:3139–45.

56. Hao CM, Yull F, Blackwell T, et al. Dehydration activates an NF-κ B-driven, COX2-dependent survival mechanism in renal medullary interstitial cells. J Clin Invest 2000;106:973–82.

57. Vadivel N, Trikudanathan S, Singh AK. Analgesic nephropathy. Kidney Int 2007; 72(4):517–20.

58. Mackinnon B, Boulton-Jones M, McLaughlin K. Analgesic-associated nephropathy in the West of Scotland: a 12-year observational study. Nephrol Dial Transplant 2003;18(9):1800.

59. Kramer HJ, Glänzer K, Düsing R. Role of prostaglandins in the regulation of renal water excretion. Kidney Int 1981;19(6):851.

60. Clark BA, Shannon RP, Rosa RM, et al. Increased susceptibility to thiazide-induced hyponatremia in the elderly. J Am Soc Nephrol 1994;5(4):1106.

61. Schlondorff D. Renal complications of nonsteroidal anti-inflammatory drugs. Kidney Int 1993;44(3):643.

62. Campbell WB. Attenuation of angiotensin II- and III-induced aldosterone release by prostaglandin synthesis inhibitors. J Clin Invest 1979;64(6):1552.

63. Ng JL, Morgan DJR, Loh NKM, et al. Life-threatening hypokalaemia associated with ibuprofen-induced renal tubular acidosis. Med J Aust 2011;194(6):313–6.

64. Soriano J. Renal tubular acidosis: the clinical entity. J Am Soc Nephrol 2002;13: 2160–70.

65. Zimran A, Kramer M, Plaskin M, et al. Incidence of hyperkalaemia induced by indomethacin in a hospital population. Br Med J (Clin Res Ed) 1985; 291(6488):107.

66. DuBose TD, McDonald GA. Renal tubular acidosis. In: DuBose TD, Hamm LL, editors. Acid-base and electrolyte disorders: a companion to Brenner and Rector's the kidney. Philadelphia: Saunders; 2002. p. 189–206.

67. White W. Cardiovascular effects of the cyclooxygenase inhibitors. Hypertension 2007;49:408–18.

68. Struthers AD, Unger T. Physiology of aldosterone and pharmacology of aldosterone blockers. Eur Heart J Suppl 2011;13(Suppl B):B27–30.

69. Izhar M, Alausa T, Folker A, et al. Effects of COX inhibition on blood pressure and kidney function in ACE inhibitor-treated blacks and Hispanics. Hypertension 2004;43:574–7.

70. Whelton A, SUCCESS-VII Investigators. Effects of celecoxib and rofecoxib on blood pressure and edema in patients >65 years of age with systemic hypertension and osteoarthritis. Am J Cardiol 2002;90:959–63.

71. Houston MC, Weir M, Gray J, et al. The effects of nonsteroidal anti-inflammatory drugs on blood pressures of patients with hypertension controlled by verapamil. Arch Intern Med 1995;155:1049–54.

72. Klassen DK, Jane LH, Young DY, et al. Assessment of blood pressure during naproxen therapy in hypertensive patients treated with nicardipine. Am J Hypertens 1995;8:146–53.

73. Sowers JR, Celecoxib Rofecoxib Efficacy and Safety in Comorbidities Evaluation Trial (CRESCENT) Investigators. The effects of cyclooxygenase-2 inhibitors and nonsteroidal antiinflammatory therapy on 24-hour blood pressure in patients

with hypertension, osteoarthritis and type 2 diabetes. Arch Intern Med 2005;165: 161–8.

74. Johnson AG, Nguyen TV, Day RO. Do nonsteroidal anti-inflammatory drugs affect blood pressure? A meta-analysis. Ann Intern Med 1994;121:289–300.

75. Julius S, Kjeldsen SE, Weber M, et al, VALUE Trial Group. Outcomes in hypertensive patients at high CV risk treated with regimens based on valsartan or amlodipine: the VALUE randomised trial. Lancet 2004;19(363):2022–31.

76. Graham DJ, Campen D, Hui R, et al. Risk of acute myocardial infarction and sudden cardiac death in patients treated with cyclo-oxygenase 2 selective and non-selective non-steroidal anti-inflammatory drugs: nested case-control study. Lancet 2005;365:475–81.

Diagnosis and Evaluation of Renal Cysts

Jack Waterman, DO[a,b,*]

KEYWORDS

- Simple renal cysts • Complex renal cysts
- Autosomal-dominant polycystic kidney disease • Acquired cystic kidney disease

KEY POINTS

- Simple renal cysts are common findings and have specific imaging criteria that render them a benign condition. When these criteria are not met, and the cyst has a complex appearance, further evaluation with enhanced imaging studies becomes necessary to exclude the presence of malignancy.
- Renal cysts may be associated with reduced renal function, reduced renal size, and hypertension. Therefore their presence warrants screening for underlying kidney disease.
- Acquired cystic kidney disease is well documented in patients with advanced chronic kidney disease and is associated with an increased risk of renal malignancy. Patients with this disorder should be followed intermittently for the development of renal cell carcinoma.
- Differentiating between multicystic, polycystic, and acquired cystic kidney disease occasionally presents a challenge in clinical practice. Certain characteristics will help to distinguish these patients, and often chronologic assessment is necessary.

INTRODUCTION

Renal cysts are the most common structural lesions of the kidneys and represent a diverse group of entities, each having their unique significance. With the widespread use of diagnostic imaging studies, the incidental finding of renal cysts has become a frequent clinical dilemma for patients and their treating physicians. Often regarded as insignificant, there are concerns that would prompt further diagnostic evaluation and need for follow-up. This article focuses on issues pertaining to the more common adult cystic diseases including simple and complex renal cysts, autosomal-dominant polycystic kidney disease (ADPKD) and acquired cystic kidney disease (ACKD). Several points will be emphasized:

- The evaluation of solitary renal cysts for their malignant potential

Disclosures: None.
[a] College of Osteopathic Medicine, Nova Southeastern University, 3301 College Avenue, Fort Lauderdale, FL 33314, USA; [b] Jupiter Kidney Center, 1701 North Military Trail, #140, Jupiter, FL 33458, USA
* Jupiter Kidney Center, 1701 North Military Trail, #140, Jupiter, FL 33458.
E-mail address: Renal@me.com

- Possible implications of simple renal cysts as potential associated risk factors for underlying renal disease
- The association of ACKD with chronic kidney disease and the risk of malignancy
- Distinguishing multicystic disease from polycystic kidney disease and ACKD

CLASSIFICATION OF CYSTIC DISORDERS

It is imperative to have a classification scheme to provide a framework for the various cystic disorders given their diversity in regard to anatomy, multiplicity, genetics, and clinical presentation. William Osler in the Principles and Practice of Medicine described 3 varieties of cysts: (1) The small cyst described in connection with chronic nephritis (2) solitary cysts and (3) congenital cystic kidneys.[1] After more than a century, the general concept is much the same. However, there are various ways to consider the different cystic disorders.

Anatomic location is one way of differentiating cystic disease. Much of the understanding about the genesis of cysts has been achieved through microdissection studies, localizing cysts to specific nephron segments.[2] Most cysts arise from tubular epithelial cells.[3] Others may arise differently, as with peripelvic cysts, which emanate from lymphatic channels. Cysts may have a predominance in the cortex, while in other conditions they localize in the medullary region as is the case with medullary cystic disease.

Cysts may be solitary or multiple. This would be a distinguishing factor separating simple renal cysts from a disorder such as polycystic kidney disease.

The course of cystic disease may be variable. Some disorders rarely affect renal function, while others have a hallmark trait that leads to progressive renal failure. Some disorders are localized to the kidney, while others behave as a systemic disease process.

Classification of renal cysts therefore must incorporate anatomic, clinical, and genetic information.[3] Despite all of these variables, some classification schemes group cystic diseases as either hereditary, developmental, or acquired. Fick and Gabow have categorized cysts accordingly as reflected and modified in **Table 1**.[4]

Table 1
Classification of cystic diseases of the kidneys

Genetic	Acquired	Developmental
Autosomal-dominant		
ADPKD	Simple renal cysts	Medullary sponge kidney
Tuberous sclerosis complex	Parapelvic and peripelvic cysts	Multicystic dysplasia
Von Hippel-Lindau disease	Multilocular cystic nephroma	Pyelocalyceal cysts
Medullary cystic disease	Hypokalemic cystic disease	
	ACKD	
	Renal cystic neoplasms	
Autosomal-recessive		
Autosomal-recessive polycystic kidney disease		
Juvenile nephronophthisis		
Cysts associated with multiple malformation syndromes		

Data from Fick GM, Gabow PA. Hereditary and acquired cystic disease of the kidney. Kidney Int 1994;46:952; and Torres VE, Grantam JJ. Cystic diseases of the kidney. Brenner and Rector's the kidney. 8th edition. Philadelphia: Saunders; 2008. p. 1429.

This article will focus on 3 primary disorders, namely simple renal cysts, ADPKD, and ACKD. A few other diseases also merit comment given their occurrence in the adult population.

Tuberous sclerosis complex is an autosomal-dominant disorder that affects multiple organs including the skin, central nervous system, and kidney. Skin manifestations include hypomelanotic macules and facial angiofibromas. Central nervous system (CNS) findings include cortical tubers and seizures. Renal manifestations include cysts, angiomyolipomas, and an increased frequency of renal malignancies. Renal failure may occur in this syndrome.

Von Hippel-Lindau disease is another dominantly transmitted disease associated with renal cysts and a high incidence of renal cell carcinoma, which may be multiple and bilateral. Other characteristics include retinal hemangiomas, cerebellar and spinal hemangioblastomas, pheochromocytomas, endocrine pancreatic tumors, and epididymal cystadenomas. Metastatic renal cell carcinoma is the leading cause of death.

Medullary cystic disease also has an autosomal-dominant pattern of transmission and is associated with small cysts at the corticomedullary junction. Tubular atrophy and interstitial fibrosis are common as well as progressive loss of renal function. Patients commonly develop polydipsia and polyuria, and there is an association with gout.

Medullary sponge kidney is a developmental disorder characterized by tubular dilatation of the collecting ducts and gives the radiographic appearance of nephrocalcinosis. This disorder is not uncommonly asymptomatic, although may be associated with renal-concentrating defects, calculi, and recurrent urinary tract infections. Mild renal dysfunction may occur, although it is rare to see end-stage renal disease (ESRD) as a consequence of this entity.

Parapelvic and peripelvic renal cysts are grouped together, since they are often used interchangeably. O'Neill points out that parapelvic cysts are parenchymal in origin and protrude into the renal sinus, while peripelvic cysts are dilated lymphatic channels that are common after the fourth decade. They may distort the renal sinus and calices being confused with a hydronephrotic process, but rarely cause true obstruction.[3,5]

SIMPLE RENAL CYSTS

Simple renal cysts are the most frequently encountered cystic lesions of the kidney.

They may be solitary or multiple in nature. William Osler describes solitary renal cysts in the Principles and Practice of Medicine published in 1892. The text reads as follows: "Solitary cysts ranging in size from a marble to an orange or even larger, are occasionally found in kidneys which present no other changes. They never give rise to symptoms, though in exceptional cases, they may form tumors of considerable size."[1]

Simple renal cysts are solitary, unilateral, and cortical 70% to 80% of the time[2] and typically extend outside of the renal parenchyma. The cysts are usually lined by a single layer of epithelial cells and are filled with a fluid that is similar to an ultrafiltrate of plasma.[3]

The cysts may arise from tubular epithelium as a consequence of cell proliferation. Microdissection studies reveal diverticula of the distal convoluted collecting tubule and collecting duct that increase with age. After progressive dilation, these detach from the nephron, forming cysts that continue to demonstrate turnover of cyst fluid.[3] There also may be a weakening of the tubular basement membrane in the formation of the distal nephron diverticula.[6]

Cysts tend to increase in incidence with age (**Fig. 1**).[2,6] Although the incidence is variable, data compiled from autopsy results and imaging studies show a frequency of up to 50% in adults over the age of 50.[7] There is a 2:1 male predominance. Cysts are rare under the age of 30.[8] When present at that age, they should raise a concern for the expression of an underlying genetic disorder.[5]

Cysts may increase in size with time. In evaluating the 10-year natural history of simple cysts, Terada and colleagues found that the rate of progression was 1.6 mm/y or an increment in cyst size of 3.9% per year. It was rare for cysts to more than double their size. Cysts tend to grow more rapidly in younger individuals and slow with older age. Multilocular cysts were more likely to increase in size.[2,9]

The risk factors for the development of renal cysts are reported to be older age, male gender, renal dysfunction, hypertension, and smoking.[2,9] The interesting association between hypertension, renal dysfunction, and renal cysts raises an interesting question regarding the pathophysiology. Could it be that renal cysts are a biomarker for underlying renal pathology? Several studies have looked at the association of cystic disease with reduced renal size, reduced renal function, and hypertension.

Al-Said and O'Neill reviewed 2526 renal ultrasounds of which 385 had 1 or more cysts. In this population, there were 82 solitary kidneys. There was an association of renal cysts and reduced renal size, implying a reduction in nephron mass. Additionally, there was an increased association of cysts in patients with solitary kidneys, again implying evidence for a causative role of reduced renal mass.[10] Similarly, a study evaluating 561 hospitalized patients under the age of 60 by Al-Said and colleagues[8] found that there was an association of reduced renal function in patients with renal cysts as measured by estimated creatinine clearance, raising the question that there is a linkage between the development of cysts and underlying renal disease. The postulate is raised that nephron loss leads to aberrant growth of remaining tubular structures, leading to tubular dilatation and ultimate cyst formation. Rule and colleagues[11] evaluated 1957 consecutive potential kidney donors at the Mayo Clinic using contrast computed tomography (CT) and concluded that cysts greater than 5 mm may be an early marker of occult kidney disease, because they were associated with albuminuria, hyperfiltration, and hypertension.[12] Additional studies have also supported the association of renal cysts with hypertension.[13,14]

Cysts are usually asymptomatic, but if exceptionally large, they may cause flank discomfort, abdominal pain, hypertension, and hematuria. A large cyst could cause

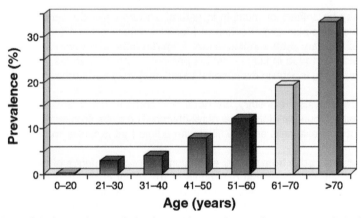

Fig. 1. Age-related prevalence of simple renal cysts. (*From* Eknoyan G. A clinical view of simple and complex renal cysts. J Am Soc Nephrol 2009;20:1874–6; with permission.)

obstructive symptoms if it was proximate to the renal pelvis. Symptoms should always raise the suspicion for an associated malignancy.[2]

The ideal imaging study for simple cysts is ultrasonography. Findings will typically reveal a round or ovoid appearance, sharply demarcated and smooth walls and a lack of internal echoes. There should be good sound wave transmission and strong posterior wall acoustic enhancement. Other imaging studies may be utilized in the evaluation simple cysts. CT and magnetic resonance imaging (MRI) have the ability to detect cysts of smaller sizes. By CT, the cyst content will typically be -10 to 20 Hounsfield units, similar to water. Cysts that develop hemorrhage or infection or have increased proteinacious content may have increased density on CT. There should not be enhancement after injection of intravenous (IV) contrast.[15] In this setting, the likelihood of malignancy is negligible (**Fig. 2**).

COMPLEX RENAL CYSTS

Cysts that do not meet the criteria for simple cysts are referred to as complex cysts. Cysts that develop septations, wall thickening, and irregularity and demonstrate calcifications should always raise the concern for malignancy and therefore need to be further evaluated. The more unusual or complex a lesion appears the higher the risk of malignancy. Lesions that appear complex deserve to be further evaluated with contrast CT or MRI. Chronologic assessment with prior studies naturally would prove invaluable.

Renal cell carcinoma comprises 2% to 3% of all cancers in the United States.[16] Cystic renal cell carcinomas represent 5% to 7% of all renal tumors.[7] The current focus is how to stratify complex cystic lesions to formulate an action plan to deal appropriately with threatening lesions and avoid unnecessary procedures. Care of patients with these lesions often falls to urology colleagues, but nephrologists and primary care providers frequently encounter these lesions and need to have an awareness of their importance and participate in the decision-making process.

A classification system was devised by Bosniak in 1986[17] and was later modified in 2003[2] to distinguish between various grades of complex cystic lesions in order to assess the risk of malignancy (**Table 2**). This system relies on the use of enhanced CT scanning. The variables utilized include thickening of the cyst wall, septations,

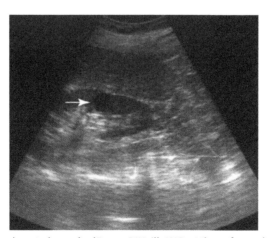

Fig. 2. Simple renal cyst (*arrow*). (*From* O'Neill WC. Atlas of renal ultrasonography. Philadelphia: Saunders; 2001. p. 82.)

Table 2
Bosniak classification system

Bosniak Category	Features
I	Thin cyst wall, does not contain septae, calcification, or solid components; does not enhance with contrast
II	Minimal regular thickening of the cyst wall, few hairline septae; fine calcification may be present in the cyst wall or septae; does not enhance with contrast
IIf	Minimal thickening of the cyst wall and septae, increased number of thin septae; calcifications may be nodular or thick. Minimal enhancement of a hairline thin septum or wall; however, no enhancing soft tissue elements; well marginated; nonenhancing high attenuation totally intrarenal lesions >3 cm included
III	Irregular thickened walls or septae, irregular calcifications; elements show enhancement
IV	Grossly irregular thickening of cyst wall and septae with irregular calcifications; clearly enhancing

Adapted from McGuire BB, Fitzpatrick JM. The diagnosis and management of complex renal cysts. Curr Opin Urol 2010;20:349–54.

calcification, nodularity, and the presence or absence of tissue enhancement. Benign cysts should not enhance with contrast, because they are avascular and do not directly communicate with the nephron.[15]

Cysts are determined to be in 1 of 5 categories based on their appearance. Lesions in Bosniak categories I and II are generally benign and would require only periodic follow-up. Bosniak category IV lesions carry an 85% to 100% risk of malignancy and require surgical intervention. Bosniak IIf and III lesions are less predictable and warrant further evaluation and follow-up to exclude malignancy. Class III lesions have a 40% to 60% chance of malignancy.[2] There are several different pathologic lesions that may comprise these neoplasms, including cystic clear cell carcinoma, multilocular cystic renal cell carcinoma, cystic nephroma, and mixed epithelial and stromal tumors (**Fig. 3**).[18]

Indeterminate lesions that do not meet criteria for simple cysts or cystic neoplasms (class IIf and III) comprise approximately 8% of renal cysts.[7] Any complex lesion deserves follow-up with an enhanced modality, namely contrast-enhanced CT or enhanced MRI. Different practitioners may have different preferences based on their experience, and naturally each patient's case should be individualized. MRI may complement CT findings but is not always necessarily superior to CT. In fact, MRI has been reported to be compatible with the Bosniak classification scheme, although it might upgrade type IIf lesions, since MRI may be more sensitive in detection of septae and enhancement. MRI may not detect calcification; however, this is likely not a major concern.[19] Clearly MRI has the advantage of saving radiation exposure in individuals undergoing repeated studies. It would seem prudent to be consistent with the chosen modality on repeated studies, in order to be able to compare similar images. An additional modality that has gained interest is contrast-enhanced ultrasound. This study utilizes the injection of microbubbles and subtraction imaging techniques. Caution must be exercised in patients with chronic obstructive pulmonary disease (COPD) and class IV congestive heart failure (CHF) when using this modality.[20]

Biopsy of cystic renal lesions has remained an area of controversy. Previous bias against biopsy was directed at the perception of low yield and complications of tumor seeding and hemorrhage. Many clinicians are comfortable with close radiographic

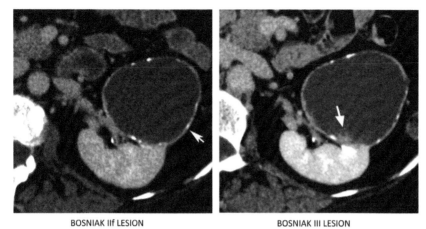

BOSNIAK IIf LESION   BOSNIAK III LESION

Fig. 3. Enhanced CT images in the same patient 6 months apart demonstrating progression in complex appearance. The arrow in the first panel shows thickened partially calcified wall. *Arrow* in the second panel shows ill-defined soft tissue enhancement. (*From* Smith AD, Remer EM, Cox KL, et al. Bosniak category IIf and III cystic renal lesions: outcomes and associations. Radiology 2012:262(1):152–60; with permission.)

surveillance of indeterminate lesions, since lack of change is a favorable sign, and increasing size or change in character would prompt intervention. Nonetheless, there are circumstances in which biopsy would prove helpful prior to committing a patient to surgical intervention.[7]

In general, lesions that appear suspicious with evidence of increased size (greater than 3 cm), lobularity, irregularity, nodularity, and measureable dye enhancement should be approached from a surgical standpoint. These would correlate to definite class III and IV lesions. Class IIf and indeterminate class III lesions should be followed at intervals, perhaps at 3 months, 6 months, and 12 months if they remain stable, and then every 6 to 12 months thereafter. Although likely benign class I and II lesions are best followed initially for the first 2 to 3 years, especially when cyst diameters are greater than 3 cm.[2] Naturally, complex lesions should have urologic evaluation and follow-up on a routine basis.

AUTOSOMAL POLYCYSTIC KIDNEY DISEASE

ADPKD is the most common hereditary kidney disease and accounts for 5% of the ESRD population worldwide.[21] It is characterized by the development of renal cysts of varying sizes and consequent enlargement of kidney as well as progressive loss of kidney function. Evidence of declining GFR occurs after the development of renal cysts, and may ultimately lead to renal failure by late middle age. Not every patient with this diagnosis reaches ESRD. Several studies have shown that only 50% of patients developed ESRD by 60 years of age.[4]

ADPKD is inherited as an autosomal-dominant trait with complete penetrance. Therefore the chance of inheritance from a parent is 50%. Mutations of 2 genes account for the vast majority of ADPKD cases. Mutation of the PKD 1 gene, which exists on chromosome 16 and encodes for polycystin1, accounts for 85% of PKD cases. Mutation of the PKD 2 gene on chromosome 4, which encodes for polycystin 2, accounts for the remainder of cases. There are some patients who cannot be localized to either locus, and this suggests either the existence of a PKD3 gene or the development of a spontaneous mutation.

Polycystins are glycoproteins involved in renal tubular development. Alterations in polycystins may account for the phenotypic expression of PKD, because they are involved with cellular proliferation, net fluid secretion, abnormal extracellular matrix, and cell–cell interactions. Abnormal polycystin function secondary to mutations leads to cyst formation through loss of mechanical cues in tubular epithelial cells that regulate tissue morphogenesis.[21] Polycystins are associated with the primary cilium of kidney tubular epithelial cells, and abnormalities may result in impaired mechano- and chemosensation that ultimately impact on cellular calcium flux. Also there may be a link to other factors contributing to cyst formation such as generation of cyclic adenosine monophosphate (cAMP), Cl-dependent fluid secretion and regulation of mTOR (mammalian target of rapamycin).[3] All of these issues have potential implication for future therapeutic intervention.

Patients with PKD1 generally have a more severe course with earlier onset of disease as well as more rapid decline of renal function than PKD2. They are also more likely to have substantial extrarenal manifestations of cystic disease such as liver cysts, cysts in other organs, aneurysms, valvular heart issues, and diverticuli. Complications of PKD include hypertension, cyst hemorrhage, cyst infection, pain, and nephrolithiasis. Notably there is a minor incidence of intracranial aneurysms, which could rarely lead to cerebral hemorrhage. PKD2 patients generally have a less aggressive course with later onset of detection and development of renal failure. Studies have shown that PKD1 patients developed ESRD approximately 15 years earlier than patients with PKD2.[21,22]

Although molecular genetic testing including both DNA linkage analysis and gene-based mutation screening can be performed, the most convenient way to screen for ADPKD is ultrasonography. Ultrasound is affordable, portable, noninvasive, and avoids radiation exposure. The typical PKD kidney is enlarged and demonstrates numerous bilateral cysts of varying size. Liver cysts along with cystic involvement of other organs may be evident also.

Ravine described the original ultrasound criteria for establishing a diagnosis of PKD. Original criteria centered on the establishment of a diagnosis in the setting of a PKD1 genotype. Later, an international consortium of PKD experts established unified criteria for the diagnosis, which encompass those with an unknown genotype although at risk given their family history.[21–23] Because genotype is seldom definitively known, in the usual clinical setting the unified criteria offer a convenient approach.

Criteria for at-risk individuals (indicating a family history) with an unknown genotype are reflected as follows. In individuals between the age group of 15 to 39 years of age, at least 3 unilateral or bilateral cysts must be present. In individuals 40 to 59 years of age at least 2 cysts in each kidney are required. Individuals older than 60 years of age require 4 cysts in each kidney. Increase in renal size, although a hallmark of PKD, has not yet been included in the criteria. An ultrasound with 0 or 1 cyst at the age of 40 years virtually excludes the diagnosis of ADPKD in at-risk individuals.[23] As stated previously, the presence of a renal cyst under the age of 30 should raise the concern for the development of a multicystic disorder (**Fig. 4**, **Table 3**).

These criteria become important in counseling individuals for family planning and in screening donors for organ donation. Additional testing in these patients may be necessary, such as utilization of contrast CT, MRI or genetic testing. Generally, screening for PKD does not begin before the age of 18 years. The consequences of screening should be discussed at length with the patient and concerned family members.

The renal complications of PKD include nephrolithiasis, hemorrhage, cyst infection, malignancy, cyst rupture, and obstruction. Nephrolithiasis can occur in 16% to 25% of

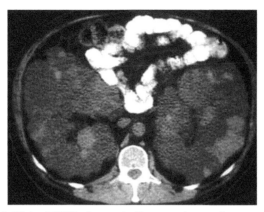

Fig. 4. Noncontrast CT in ADPKD demonstrating massive nephromegaly with numerous bilateral cysts. (*From* Chapman AB. Autosomal dominant polycystic kidney disease: time for a change? J Am Soc Nephrol 2007;18(5):1399–407.)

ADPKD patients. Although ultrasound may be utilized in the evaluation of stones, CT is a superior modality in this setting. Complex cysts frequently appear in PKD and may be secondary to cyst hemorrhage or infection. CT and MRI are both useful in this setting to better characterize the abnormality. Positron emission tomography (PET) scanning may be useful in cases in which there is suspicion of infection, because infected cysts may be flourodeoxyglucose avid. Malignancy, particularly renal cell carcinoma, may occur in ADPKD patients, but there is no definitive association as there is with von Hippel-Lindau disease. Because repeated evaluations may be necessary in the case of complex cysts, MRI may be a better modality to avoid excessive radiation exposure and nephrotoxic effects of IV contrast. There has been considerable concern regarding the use of gadolinium in the setting of CKD given the risk of nephrogenic systemic fibrosis. If the more stable forms of gadolinium are utilized, there may be less of risk of this feared complication.[23]

Several factors may be responsible for the observed decline in renal function associated with ADPKD. The Consortium for Radiologic Imaging Studies of Polycystic Kidney Disease cohort (CRISP consortium) was designed by the National Institutes of Health (NIH) to assess whether total kidney volume could predict future renal impairment. In fact, total kidney volume assessed by MRI has strong predictive power in the determination of progression of renal failure compared with other variables.[23,24]

Table 3	
Autosomal-dominant polycystic kidney disease criteria for at risk patients with unknown genotype	
Age in Years	**Number of Cysts**
15–39	At least 3 unilateral or bilateral
40–59	At least 2 cysts in each kidney
>60	At least 4 cysts in each kidney

Data from Rahbari-Oskoui F, Mittal A, Mittal P, et al. Renal relevant radiology: radiologic imaging in autosomal-dominant polycystic kidney disease. Clin J Am Soc Nephrol 2014;9:406–15.

ACQUIRED CYSTIC KIDNEY DISEASE

ACKD develops in individuals with progressive renal disorders who have no underlying history of hereditary cystic disease. Although appreciated in the 19th century as noted by Simon in 1847 and Osler in his textbook of medicine, Dunhill reintroduced this entity in 1977. The entity was felt by Dunhill to manifest as a consequence of hemodialysis.[25] It is now known that cysts develop in kidneys affected by all renal diseases and also become evident in the pre-ESRD population.

There is no agreement as to the extent of cystic change that is required for the diagnosis of ACKD. CT scanning will show evidence of numerous bilateral cysts of varying sizes. Generally, more than 1 to 5 cysts per kidney give a comfort level for the diagnosis. Most cysts will range between 0.5 and 3 cm in diameter. There seems to be a male-over-female predominance and a higher incidence in blacks.[3,4] The incidence of ACKD is shown in **Table 4**.

Both kidneys are involved in the cystic process. The kidneys are typically small or normal in size. On occasion, large cysts and increased renal size may occur. Cysts are generally smaller than in patients with ADPKD. Cysts generally do not occur in in other organs as in ADPKD (**Fig. 5**).

Patients are typically asymptomatic. Complications of cysts can occur including hemorrhage, hematuria, and flank pain. As with ADPKD, which can cause erythrocytosis, so a rising hematocrit has been seen in patients with ACKD.

Although the exact etiology of ACKD is uncertain and probably multifactorial, it has been postulated that the disease process in some regard may be instigated by systemic toxins in the uremic milieu. This is supported by the fact that cysts have been demonstrated to regress after successful renal transplantation.[15,26] This finding is not universal, and ACKD may persist in native kidneys, remaining a risk factor for neoplasia.

The most worrisome complication of ACKD is the propensity for the development of renal cell carcinoma. The reason for this predilection may be related to cystic epithelial cell proliferation, which then potentially creates the substrate for oncogenes to cause malignant transformation.[27] In the dialysis population, the incidence of renal cell carcinoma is significantly greater than the general population. The associated malignancy may be multicentric and seems to have a lower risk of metastasis than other populations with renal cell carcinomas.[3]

Given the higher incidence of renal cell carcinoma in this population, it would seem prudent to perform imaging studies on dialysis patients 3 years after 3 initiating therapy, and then every 1 to 2 years subsequent to documenting the development of cystic disease. Less clear is the optimal time for screening patients who are in the pre-ESRD population. It is this author's practice to screen patients at least every

Table 4 Incidence of acquired cystic disease	
Creatinine/Duration on Dialysis	**% Incidence**
Serum creatinine >3 mg/dL	7–22
Dialysis duration of 2 y	35
Dialysis duration of 2–4 y	58
Dialysis duration of 4–8 y	75
Dialysis duration >8 y	92

Data from Torres VE, Grantam JJ. Cystic diseases of the kidney. Brenner and Rector's the kidney. 8th edition. Philadelphia: Saunders; 2008.

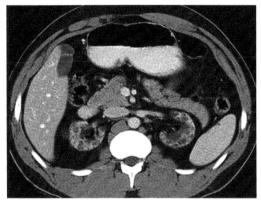

Fig. 5. Acquired cystic kidney disease demonstrating small kidneys with bilateral cysts in the setting of advanced chronic kidney disease. (*From* Chapman AB. Autosomal dominant polycystic kidney disease: time for a change? J Am Soc Nephrol 2007;18(5):1399–407.)

3 years who have no documented history of renal cystic disease, and to screen more frequently those who do manifest cysts. The author will usually screen with ultrasound and then move on to CT scanning or MRI should there be a concern for complex cystic change.

DIFFERENTIATING BETWEEN MULTICYSTIC, POLYCYSTIC, AND ACQUIRED RENAL CYSTIC DISEASE

Differentiating between multicystic, polycystic, and ACKD is a common dilemma in clinical nephrology practice. Often the patient must be followed over time in order to make this distinction.

Those patients with multiple simple renal cysts will tend to be older, have better glomerular filtration rates on detection, and be less likely to have significant progression of renal failure. In general, there is lack of a family history of renal cystic disease. Kidney size will typically be in the normal range. Associated cysts are not found in other organs. The incidence of hypertension is variable.

Patients with ADPKD will tend to be younger on initial detection of their cysts and usually have a family history of renal cystic disease. Cysts are often innumerable and of varying sizes. Kidney function tends to deteriorate over time, and kidney size is notably increased. Cysts may be present in other organs along with other systemic comorbid findings as previously discussed. Hypertension is common.

ACKD will present in those individuals who have more advanced renal failure. Renal size will tend to be reduced. Cyst size is usually not excessive. There is lack of association with cysts in other organs. The incidence of hypertension would be expected to be higher in this population. This group of patients needs to be monitored closely for the development of renal malignancy.

SUMMARY

Renal cysts are commonly encountered in clinical practice and deserve scrutiny in order to avoid overlooking a significant disease process. Though most cysts found incidentally on routine imaging studies will prove to be benign simple cysts, there must be an index of suspicion for the potential of a neoplastic process and also for the association with a multicystic disease.

Fortunately with the imaging modalities currently available, the majority of cystic disorders can be diagnosed confidently and followed for any sinister change. Concomitant systemic issues should be correlated with the finding of renal cysts to exclude a genetic syndrome, and renal function studies should be monitored to assess for any degree of loss of renal function.

The issues that face clinicians routinely were presented to heighten the awareness of the significance of renal cystic disease and focus on a few salient points:

- Simple renal cysts are common findings and have specific imaging criteria that render them a benign condition. When these criteria are not met and the cyst has a complex appearance, further evaluation with enhanced imaging studies becomes necessary to exclude the presence of malignancy. The Bosniak classification system was devised to assist in this process. High-grade lesions and certainly those that enhance with contrast are highly suspicious and require urologic assessment and ultimately may require surgical intervention.
- Studies have focused on the association of simple cysts with underlying renal disease. The question of whether cysts are a biomarker of occult renal dysfunction has been raised. Suffice it to say that several studies have focused on the association of cystic disease with reduced renal function, reduced renal size, albuminuria, and hypertension. This remains an interesting area for further research.
- ACKD has been reported for well over a century and is known to be associated with an increased risk of renal cancer in the dialysis population. There is evidence that ACKD begins in the pre-ESRD population. Although cystic changes have been shown to regress with transplantation, this group remains at high risk for the development of neoplasia. All patients with this diagnosis need to be under continuing surveillance.
- Finally, clinicians are asked to render a specific diagnosis in patients with multiple cysts and determine if they have simple cystic disease, ADPKD, or ACKD. On occasion, the situation is unclear but can be answered with obtaining a detailed family history, assessing renal function, and scrutinizing imaging studies. Attention to renal size, searching for cysts in other organs, and appreciating other co-morbidities are key elements to aid in distinguishing these entities. On occasion it is necessary to follow the evolution of the disease process over time to solve the puzzle.

REFERENCES

1. Osler MD. The principles and practice of medicine. New York: D. Appleton and Company; 1892. p. 772.
2. Eknoyan G. A clinical view of simple and complex renal cysts. J Am Soc Nephrol 2009;20:1874–6.
3. Torres VE, Grantham JJ. Cystic diseases of the kidney. In: Brenner BM, editor. Brenner and Rector's the kidney. 8th edition. Philadelphia: W.B. Saunders; 2008. p. 1428–62.
4. Fick GM, Gabow PA. Hereditary and acquired cystic disease of the kidney. Kidney Int 1994;46:951–64.
5. O'Neill WC. Atlas of renal ultrasonography. Philadelphia: W.B. Saunders; 2001. p. 99.
6. Terada N, Ichioka K, Matsuta Y, et al. The natural history of simple renal cysts. J Urol 2002;167:21–3.
7. McGuire BB, Fitzpatrick JM. The diagnosis and management of complex renal cysts. Curr Opin Urol 2010;20:349–54.

8. Al-Said J, Brumback MA, Moghazi S, et al. Reduced renal function in patients with simple renal cysts. Kidney Int 2004;65:2303–8.
9. Terada N, Arai Y, Kinukawa N, et al. The 10-year natural history of simple renal cysts. Urology 2008;71:7–11.
10. Al-Said J, O'Neill WC. Reduced kidney size in patients with simple renal cysts. Kidney Int 2003;64:1059–64.
11. Rule AD, Sasiwimonphan, K, Lieske JC, et al. Characteristics of renal cystic and solid lesions based on contrast-enhanced computed tomography of potential kidney donors. Am J Kidney Dis 2012;59(5):611–8.
12. Grantham JJ. Solitary renal cysts: worth a second look? Am J Kidney Dis 2012;59(5):593–4.
13. Chin HJ, Ro H, Lee HJ, et al. The clinical significances of simple renal cyst: is it related to hypertension or renal dysfunction? Kidney Int 2006;70:1468–73.
14. Lee YJ, Kim MS, Cho S, et al. Association between simple renal cysts and development of hypertension in healthy middle-aged men. J Hypertens 2012;30:700–4.
15. Glassberg KI. Renal dysgenesis and cystic disease of the kidney. In: Welsh P, editor. Campbell's urology. 8th edition. Philadelphia: W.B. Saunders; 2002. p. 1937–94.
16. Bonsib SM. Renal cystic diseases and renal neoplasms: a mini-review. Clin J Am Soc Nephrol 2009;4:1998–2007.
17. Bosniak MA. The current radiological approach to renal cysts. Radiology 1986;158:1–10.
18. Smith AD, Remer EM, Cox KL, et al. Bosniak category IIF and III cystic renal lesions: outcomes and associations. Radiology 2012;262:152–60.
19. Israel G, Hindman N, Bosniak MA, et al. Evaluation of cystic renal masses: comparison of CT and MR imaging by using the bosniak classification system. Radiology 2004;231(2):365–71.
20. Ascenti G, Mazziotti S, Zimbaro G, et al. Complex cystic renal masses: characterization with contrast-enhanced US. Radiology 2007;243:158–65.
21. Pei Y, Obaji J, Dupuis A, et al. Unified criteria for ultrasonographic diagnosis of ADPKD. J Am Soc Nephrol 2009;20:205–12.
22. Pei Y. Diagnostic approach in autosomal dominant polycystic kidney disease. Clin J Am Soc Nephrol 2006;1:1108–14.
23. Rahbari-Oskoui F, Mittal A, Mittal P, et al. Renal relevant radiology: radiologic imaging in autosomal dominant polycystic kidney disease. Clin J Am Soc Nephrol 2014;9:406–15.
24. Chapman A. Autosomal dominant polycystic kidney disease: time for a change? J Am Soc Nephrol 2007;18:1399–407.
25. Dunnill MS, Millard PR, Oliver D. Acquired cystic disease of the kidneys: a hazard of long-term intermittent maintenance haemodialysis. J Clin Pathol 1977;30:868–77.
26. Grantham J. Acquired cystic kidney disease. Kidney Int 1991;40:143–52.
27. Marple JT, MacDougall M, Chonko AM. Renal cancer complicating acquired cystic kidney disease. J Am Soc Nephrol 1994;4:1951–6.

The Primary Care Physician/Nephrologist Partnership in Treating Chronic Kidney Disease

Mark D. Baldwin, DO[a,b],*

KEYWORDS

- CKD (chronic kidney disease) • Referral • Hypertension • Remnant kidney • Dialysis
- Hyperparathyroidism • Proteinuria • Albuminuria

KEY POINTS

- Chronic kidney disease (CKD) is a common disease and closely associated with diabetes mellitus and hypertension, 2 of the most common serious illness seen in a primary care physician's office.
- Cardiovascular disease and CKD share many similar pathophysiological mechanisms.
- The progression of CKD can be slowed in many cases by a number of interventions.
- Early nephrology referral can have a significant impact on the course of CKD, improve mortality and morbidity, and improve the quality of life in many cases.

INTRODUCTION

Chronic kidney disease (CKD) continues to increase in both incidence and prevalence in the United States and elsewhere.[1] Much of this can be attributed to the obesity epidemic and subsequent rise in the rates of diabetes mellitus and hypertension. A number of studies have demonstrated improved patient outcomes by early nephrology referral; but all too often, these referrals are made late in the patient's clinical course.[2–4] Early referral engages not only the nephrologist, but frequently involves other professional team members, such as a dietician, skilled in CKD to provide a comprehensive approach to the patient.

Many overt signs and symptoms, including pain, are frequently absent in all but the late stages of CKD, thus delaying the patient's perceived need to seek medical

Dr M.D. Baldwin has not received any grants, speakers fee, or other remuneration directly or indirectly related to any of the topics discussed in this article.

[a] Ohio University of Osteopathic Medicine, 3433 Alger Rd., Athens, OH, USA; [b] Private Practice, Columbus Neighborhood Health Center, 3433 Agler Rd., Suite 2800, Columbus, OH 43219, USA
* Ohio University of Osteopathic Medicine, 3433 Alger Rd., Athens, OH.
E-mail address: mdb51@earthlink.net

attention. As the early diagnosis of CKD is made by laboratory methods (ie, serum blood urea nitrogen, creatinine, proteinuria, and albuminuria), the role of the primary care physician (PCP) is essential in partnering with the nephrologist to facilitate a smooth transition in the patient's care, and also to identify potentially reversible causes of kidney dysfunction and, perhaps, slow its progression.

The impact of CKD on all-cause mortality is significant. According to the National Vital Statistics Report on causes of death in the United States for 2010, *kidney disease ranked as the eighth most common cause of death.*[5] *Diabetes mellitus, which is the most common cause of CKD in the United States, is seventh.*[5] *CKD is a significant risk factor for cardiovascular mortality, which is the leading cause of death in patients with CKD.*[6] There is increased cancer-related mortality, especially in gastrointestinal, lung, and breast tumors in patients with CKD.[7]

Many of the determinants in the progression of CKD are the same as seen in cardiovascular disease; many of the features in the treatment of cardiovascular disease will also slow the progression of CKD in many patients.[8] This suggests common underlying pathophysiological mechanism(s) at work.[9]

Until recently, terms such as chronic renal failure or chronic renal insufficiency have been used, but without any clear objective values associated with them. Although normal kidney function and end-stage renal disease (ESRD on dialysis) have been the 2 well-defined extremes of renal function, the territory between them has been nebulous and indistinct.

The National Kidney Foundation Kidney Disease Outcomes Quality Initiative (KDOQI) guidelines, published in 2002, were later revised and published by the International Society of Nephrology as the Kidney Disease Improving Global Outcomes (KDIGO) in 2005 and updated in 2012.[10–12] These guidelines established clear-cut definitions for the diagnosis of CKD, and also, based on a thorough review of evidence-based medicine, recommendations for diagnostic testing, management of complications of CKD, both renal and nonrenal. In addition, these guidelines made specific recommendations as to the timing and benefits of early nephrology referral and in the management of these patients.[12]

What Is Chronic Kidney Disease?

CKD can manifest in a number of ways, as abnormalities of protein excretion, usually in the form of albuminuria, urine sediment abnormalities (ie, red blood cell casts), electrolyte and/or acid/base abnormalities, abnormalities of structure of the kidneys or microscopic abnormalities, or a history of renal transplantation. This may or may not be associated with a *greater than 50% decline* of "normal renal function," from baseline glomerular filtration rate (GFR) of 120 mL/min/1.73 m². This is usually seen at a GFR of less than 60 mL/min/1.73 m². These must be *present for longer than 3 months* to differentiate from acute kidney injury (AKI) (**Box 1**).

CKD can be staged based on GFR and on albumin excretion (**Fig. 1**).

Evaluation and estimation of glomerular filtration rate and proteinuria

A number of formulas have developed over the years to estimate the GFR, with varying degrees of accuracy. These are based on the patient's serum creatinine, along with weight, sex, age, and/or race, depending on the formula used. *The most important factor in using any of these methods is that the renal function must be stable and not rapidly deteriorating or improving to yield the most accurate results.*[12] A serum creatinine is an estimate of renal function, but it is only a rough estimate. In addition, the classic 24-hour urine collection for creatinine clearance, which was the standard

> **Box 1**
> **Criteria for chronic kidney disease (CKD) (either of the following present for >3 months)**
>
> | Marker of kidney damage(1 or more) | Example |
> | --- | --- |
> | Albuminuria >30 mg/24 hours | Nephrotic syndrome, diabetes |
> | Urine sediment abnormalities | Red blood cell (RBC) casts, glomerulonephritis |
> | Anomalies of electrolytes and acid base | Renal tubular acidosis |
> | Structural abnormalities of histology on biopsy | Membranous nephropathy, Systemic lupus erythematosis (SLE) |
> | Structural abnormalities on imaging | Polycystic kidney disease |
> | History of renal transplantation | |
> | Decreased glomerular filtration rate (GFR) | <60 mL/min/1.73 m^2 |
>
> *From* Kidney Disease: Improving Global Outcomes (KDIGO) Work Group. KDIGO clinical practice guidelines for the evaluation and management of chronic kidney disease. Kidney Int Suppl 2013;3(1):5.

for decades, is fraught with errors in collection and inconsistency in secretion of creatinine within the tubules.

The serum creatinine represents a balance between muscle metabolism (anabolism and catabolism) and renal excretion. Any factor that influences any of the components will be reflected as a source of variance or error in the serum measurements (**Box 2**).

The Cockcroft-Gault equation is easy to use and provides a fair estimate of renal function[13]; however, its lack of accuracy limits its wide scale use. It was replaced by the Modification of Diet in Renal Disease (MDRD) equation, which takes race into

				Persistent albuminuria categories Description and range		
				A1	**A2**	**A3**
				Normal to mildly increased	Moderately increased	Severely increased
				<30 mg/g <3 mg/mmol	30–300 mg/g 3–30 mg/mmol	>300 mg/g >30 mg/mmol
GFR categories (ml/min/ 1.73 m^2) Description and range	**G1**	Normal or high	≥90		Monitor	Refer
	G2	Mildly decreased	60–89		Monitor	Refer
	G3a	Mildly to moderately decreased	45–59	Monitor	Monitor	Refer
	G3b	Moderately to severely decreased	30–44	Monitor	Monitor	Refer
	G4	Severely decreased	15–29	Refer*	Refer*	Refer
	G5	Kidney failure	<15	Refer	Refer	Refer

Fig. 1. Staging of chronic kidney disease. (*From* Kidney Disease: Improving Global Outcomes (KDIGO) Work Group. KDIGO clinical practice guidelines for the evaluation and management of chronic kidney disease. Kidney Int Suppl 2013;3(1):6.)

Box 2
Sources of errors in GFR estimation using creatinine

Non steady state: acute kidney injury (AKI)

Creatinine generation factors: racial differences, muscle mass and body size, high-protein diet, creatine supplements, muscle-wasting diseases, muscle trauma/destruction, ingestion of cooked meat

Tubular secretion of creatinine factors: trimethoprim, cimetidine, fenofibrate

Extrarenal elimination of creatinine: dialysis, decreased by inhibition of gut creatininase by antibiotics, increased by large volume losses of extracellular fluid

Higher GFR: Higher measurement error in serum creatinine and GFR

Interference in creatinine measurement: spectral interference (eg, bilirubin and some drugs), chemical interference (eg, glucose, ketones, bilirubin, some drugs)

Data from Kidney Disease: Improving Global Outcomes (KDIGO) Work Group. KDIGO clinical practice guidelines for the evaluation and management of chronic kidney disease. Kidney Int Suppl 2013;3:19–6, 39.

---

consideration in the estimate of creatinine clearance. The MDRD is adequate for a good estimate of the renal function in most patients.[14] A newer method has been developed, the Chronic Kidney Disease Epidemiology Collaboration (CKD-EPI), and is more accurate.[15] Both the MDRD and CKD-EPI were compared with patients with CKD and normal renal function undergoing [125]Iothalamate clearance as a reference comparison. The only drawback to the MRD and CKD-EPI equations are that both require an advanced calculation.

Cockcroft-Gault equation

$$\text{Creatinine Clearance} = \frac{140 - \text{age} \times \text{weight (kg)}}{72 \times \text{serum creatinine (Scr)}} \times \left(0.85 \text{ for females}\right)$$

Modification of diet in renal disease

$$175 \times \text{SCr}^{-1.154} \times \text{age}^{-0.203} \times 0.742 \text{ (if female)} \times 1.212 \text{ (if black)}$$

Chronic Kidney Disease Epidemiology Collaboration

$$\text{eGFR} = 141 \times \min(\text{Scr}/\kappa, 1)\alpha \times \max(\text{Scr}/\kappa, 1) - 1.209 \times 0.993 \text{ Age} \times 1.018$$
(if female) × 1.159 (if black)

where eGFR is the estimated GFR, Scr is serum creatinine in mg/dL, κ is 0.7 for females and 0.9 for males, α is −0.329 for females and −0.411 for males, min indicates the minimum of Scr/κ or 1, and max indicates the maximum of Scr/κ or 1.

Cystatin C

This measurement has been suggested recently as one that is more reliable than creatinine-based estimation of GFR. However, it remains to be seen if it will emerge as a preferred test to more accurately reflect the GFR in most clinical scenarios.[12]

Evaluation of proteinuria and albuminuria

Proteinuria, with or without reduction in the GFR, is an indication of significant renal damage and is in itself damaging to the tubules.[16] Quantification of protein or albumin excretion is important not only in diagnosis, but also in prognosis and monitoring of treatment efficacy.

Abnormal urinary protein excretion, usually in the form of albumin, is a common reason for referral to a nephrologist.[12] This is usually detected by a urine dipstick or an automated urinalysis. Many of the strip tests are specific for albumin, but do not detect other types of protein, such as globulins, as seen in monoclonal gammopathies. All urines should be evaluated with sulfasalicylic acid reagent, which will precipitate all proteins as a screening measure, if the reagent strips test only for albumin.[12] This helps to distinguish glomerular sources of proteinuria, which demonstrate selective albuminuria, from paraproteinemias such as myeloma, in which proteinuria originated from the overproduction of monoclonal proteins, which are nephrotoxic.

If screening tests for urine protein are positive, then quantification is done. Twenty-four-hour urine collections for total protein are no longer recommended, due to multiple error sources and difficulty in ensuring adequacy of collection.[12] It has been replaced by measuring the urine protein to urine creatinine ratio from an early morning urine sample (EMU). This value correlates to the excretion of protein in grams per day on a 24-hour collection (**Fig. 2**).[17]

For example, if the EMU protein was 240 mg/g day and the urine creatinine was 60 mg/g day,

$$\frac{240}{60} = 4$$

which would approximate 4 grams per day of protein excretion.

Because albumin is the predominant protein excreted in most clinical conditions, it also can be seen in other systemic illnesses, such as diabetes, hypertension, and cardiac and cerebrovascular diseases. Albumin also should be quantified in a similar manner as nonalbumin protein with an albumin-to-creatinine ratio (ACR). The terminology of microalbuminuria and macroalbuminuria, which has been used for many years, is now being replaced by the classification of albuminuria discussed in **Box 3**.[12]

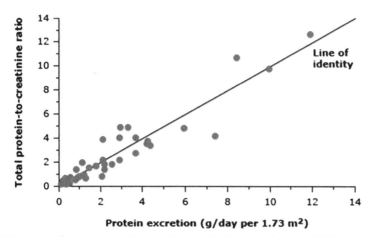

Fig. 2. Measuring the urine protein to urine creatinine ratio from an EMU sample. (*Data from* Ginsberg JM, Chang BS, Matarese RA, et al. Use of single voided urine samples to estimate quantitative proteinuria. N Engl J Med 1983;309(25):1543–6.)

Box 3
Classification of albuminuria

Category	Albumin Excretion Ratio (ACR)	Terms
A1	<30	Normal to slightly increased
A2	30–300	Moderately increased
A3	>300	Severely increased

From Kidney Disease: Improving Global Outcomes (KDIGO) Work Group. KDIGO clinical practice guidelines for the evaluation and management of chronic kidney disease. Kidney Int Suppl 2013;3:5.

Sources of error in proteinuria and factors affecting urinary albumin-to-creatinine ratio

Transient elevation in albuminuria: menstrual blood contamination, symptomatic urinary tract infection, exercise, orthostatic proteinuria, increased vascular permeability (eg, sepsis)

Individual variability: Intrinsic biologic variability, genetic variability

Preanalytic storage conditions: Degradation of albumin before analysis

Nonrenal causes of variability in creatinine excretion: Age (lower in children and older people), race (lower in white than in black people), muscle mass (eg, amputation, paraplegia, and muscular dystrophy), gender (lower in women)

Changes in creatinine excretion: AKI

Kidney disease: Improving Global Outcomes (KDIGO) Work Group. KDIGO Clinical practice guidelines for the evaluation and management of chronic kidney disease. Kidney Int Suppl 2013;3:59.

Causes of Chronic Kidney Disease

Diabetes mellitus remains the most common cause of CKD in the United States. Hypertension is the second most common cause of CKD and the most significant risk factor for progression of any form of CKD to ESRD. Polycystic kidney disease, glomerular diseases, and structural abnormalities while seen, are less common (**Box 4**).

At-risk populations

Kidney disease affects all groups, but African Americans are at considerably higher risk for CKD.[12] This population has a significantly higher incidence of hypertension. Risk factors of hypertension include lower socioeconomic status, lower birth

---

Box 4
Causes of CKD

Type 1 or 2 diabetes mellitus	Obstruction with stones, cancer, prostate causes
Hypertension	Ureteral reflux
Glomerulonephritis, nephrotic syndrome	Recurrent infection/pyelonephritis
Polycystic kidney disease	Other structural abnormalities, Alport syndrome
Chronic interstitial nephritis	After AKI

From U.S. Renal Disease Data System. USRDS 2013 annual data report atlas of chronic kidney disease and end stage renal disease in the United States. Bethesda (MD): National Institutes of Health; National Institute of Diabetes and Digestive and Kidney Diseases; 2013.

weight, salt sensitivity and high dietary sodium and lower potassium intake, less nocturnal decline in blood pressures ("dipping"), and increased body mass index.[18,19]

Recently, a mutation of the apolipoprotein L1 (*APOL 1*) gene has been found to be more common in African Americans as compared with Americans of European origins. Presence of *AOPL 1* confers immunity to *Trypanosoma brucei,* the etiologic agent of African sleeping sickness.[20] People with this gene have a much higher incidence of hypertensive nephrosclerosis and focal segmental glomerulosclerosis, two causes of CKD more common in African American than other groups.[21] Diabetic individuals with *APOL 1* have a more rapid progression of their CKD.[21] The treatment modalities and goal blood pressures in African Americans are different compared with other groups, and are detailed later in this article.

Physiologic Consequences and Compensation in Chronic Kidney Disease

In CKD, regardless of the cause, as the number of functioning nephrons decreases, the remaining nephrons are burdened with an increased work load to maintain the excretory, endocrine, and exocrine functions of the kidney.

For example, in a 70-kg man with a GFR of 60 mL/min/1.73 m^2, roughly an Scr of 2.0 mg/dL and 50% reduction in renal function, the work load of the remaining nephrons is doubled; at 30 mL/min/1.73 m^2 the work load is quadrupled.

To sustain the remaining renal function, the kidney compensates in several ways to maintain equilibrium and function. In the short term, this attempt maintains a multitude of functions, but long term, these compensatory mechanisms hasten the decline of renal function. *Increased activity of the renin-angiotensin-aldosterone system (RAAS), both locally in the kidney and systemically, and increased sympathetic nervous system activity*, play key roles in the generation and propagation of these mechanisms.[8,22]

Increased levels of angiotensin II play a key role in glomerular hypertrophy, mesangial expansion, efferent, and, to a lesser extent, afferent arteriolar vasoconstriction and mesangial contraction. These conditions lead to an increase in the glomerular capillary pressure, hyperfiltration, and proteinuria.[8,22] Angiotensin II and aldosterone also lead to increased sodium and water reabsorbtion in the tubules and increased blood volume which is subsequently delivered to the nephrone (**Fig. 3**).[23]

Under increased pressure, the glomerular capillary ruptures through the basement membrane, extruding white blood cells, platelets, complement, acute phase reactants, assorted cytokines, and other inflammatory material into the mesangium and Bowman Space, which reacts with the surrounding tissue. These materials, along with aldosterone, lead to fibrosis and sclerosis of the glomerular space, thus decreasing the available functioning nephrons and further taxing the remaining nephrons; leading to a downward spiral until end stage is reached.[23]

Any reduction in systemic blood pressure will slow the progression of CKD. However, drugs that block the RAAS give further benefit, far beyond simple blood pressure reduction, as they interrupt some of the pathophysiological mechanisms of progressive CKD.[22]

Interventions to Slow the Rate of Progression of Chronic Kidney Disease

Hypertension in chronic renal disease

Hypertension is a common feature of CKD, occurring in up to 85% of cases.[24] *The most significant factor in the progression of CKD, in most cases, centers on adequate blood pressure control.* The KDOQI guidelines recommend a systolic blood pressure (SBP) lower than 140 mm Hg and a diastolic blood pressure (DBP) lower than 90 mm Hg in

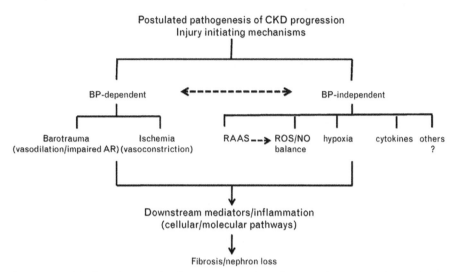

Fig. 3. Postulated pathogenesis of CKD progression. (*From* Bidani AK, Polichowski AJ, Loutzenhiser R, et al. Renal microvascular dysfunction, hypertension and CKD progression. Curr Opin Nephrol Hypertens 2013;22(1):1–9.)

diabetic and nondiabetic patients with less than 500 mg per day of albumin excretion; in diabetic and nondiabetic patients whose urinary albumin excretion is more than 500 mg per day, a goal SPB lower than 130 mm Hg and DBP lower than mm Hg is recommended.[12] In African American patients with CKD, the recommended target blood pressures are SBP lower than 130 mm Hg and DBP lower than 80 mm Hg.[25]

The causes of hypertension in patients with CKD are multifactorial. Increased activity of RAAS, increased sympathetic activity, and sodium retention, leading to volume expansion, are the most common culprits. Hence, medications directed at blunting their effect should be the cornerstone of therapy. Underlying poorly controlled essential or unrecognized secondary hypertension causes need to be fully excluded, including obstructive sleep apnea. Most nephrologists are skilled in the diagnosis and management of hypertension in patients with and without CKD (**Box 5**).

Home blood pressure measurements by the patients are not only helpful for the data they provide, but the process also engages patients in their own care, similar to home glucose monitoring in diabetes. Recommendations about the adequate sized cuff and techniques of blood pressure measurement, along with calibration with a mercury or aneroid sphygmomanometer will help to ensure adequate readings. Usually, twice-a-day readings are adequate, and more frequent measurements may be needed, if the clinical scenario dictates this (**Box 6**).

The neuroendocrine abnormalities are persistent, so must be the treatment to slow this down.

Renin-angiotensin-aldosterone inhibitors

These drugs, angiotensin-converting enzyme inhibitors (ACE-I) or angiotensin receptor blockers (ARB), should be the first medications used in most patients with diabetic or nondiabetic CKD.[12] However, their *use together is not recommended* because of lack of efficacy and increased risk of side effects.[12] Recently, aldosterone antagonists have emerged as a potential add-on therapy to reduce proteinuria and as add-on therapy for refractory hypertension.[26]

Box 5
Causative and propagating factors for hypertension in CKD

Increased activity of the renin-angiotensin-aldosterone system	Noncompliance
Increased sympathetic system activity	Obesity
Enhanced sodium retention, increased antidiuretic hormone	
Underlying hypertension: primary and undiagnosed secondary causes	
Secondary hyperparathyroidism	Obstructive sleep apnea
Medication: nonsteroidal anti-inflammatory drugs, sympathomimetics, erythropoietin	
Alcohol, illicit drugs	Excess dietary sodium
Renovascular hypertension	

These drugs lower intraglomerular pressure and decrease sodium reabsorption in the tubules. *Although there may be a transient increase in the serum creatinine, this is acceptable, as the long-term decline in renal function is much less as compared with other medications.*

There is some hesitation by some clinicians to the use of ACE-I or ARBs in patients with CKD because of concern about the transient rise in Scr. But their efficacy has been well demonstrated in diabetic and nondiabetic patients with CKD, especially in patients with CKD with proteinuria as a feature. *There is no GFR at which these medications are contraindicated,* as long as renal function, potassium levels, and blood pressures are monitored.[27]

The addition of a thiazide will augment their effectiveness, not only with blood pressure control, but also in aiding fluid mobilization. Chlorthalidone has emerged as the preferred thiazide, because of its long half-life. *Thiazides will augment the efficacy of most classes of antihypertensive medications.* Once the GFR is less than 30 mL/min per 1.73 m^2, however, thiazides are no longer indicated.[28]

Loop diuretics

This class of medication will promote fluid mobilization and natriuresis, along with blood pressure reduction. They are also indicated in the presence of edema and heart failure. *Torsemide*, which has a longer half-life, may have the potential advantage of more consistent oral absorption and longer half-life as compared with furosemide or other medication in this class.[29] Twice-a-day dosing (eg, morning and mid to late afternoon) may be needed to keep the patient in correct fluid balance. Regardless of the GFR, potassium and magnesium levels need to be regularly evaluated and replaced as needed.

Calcium channel blockers

The nondihydropyridine agents, verapamil and diltiazem, exert varying degrees of antiproteinuric effects, and should be considered as a part of blood pressure management.[30] The dihydropyridine agents (eg, amlodipine or nifedipine) do not share the antiproteinuric effect, but can be part of blood pressure management, especially in

Box 6
Goals in blood pressure control in CKD

Preservation of renal function	Decreased risk of stroke, myocardial infarction, Congestive heart failure (CHF)
Volume/sodium control	Decrease proteinuria

African American patients.[30] However, at higher doses, edema may limit their full utilization.

Aldosterone antagonists
Spironolactone and eplerenone are recommended in patients with resistant hypertension, especially with proteinuria.[31] Of course, potassium and creatinine levels need to be monitored as a part of therapy.

Adrenergic blockage agents
Although these agents do not confer any antiproteinuria benefit, certain medications of this class should be considered in certain cases of cardiac comorbidity (common condition with CKD), congestive heart failure, and overall blood pressure control. In patients with CKD, there is increased sympathetic system activity, as part of an increased neuroendocrine activity.

Older beta-blockers (propranolol, metoprolol) offer little in blood pressure reduction in resistant patients. However, combined alpha and beta blockers (ie, labetalol and carvedilol) confer good efficacy in blood pressure control.

In patients who require only once-daily medication, there is a trend to *dose these medications in the evening* to decrease the risk of early morning cardiovascular events, such as myocardial infarction or stroke.[32] As cardiovascular disease is the major cause of death in patients with CKD, this is appropriate. *It is important to understand that adequate 24-hour blood pressure control is essential to slow the progression of recommended.*

As renal function deteriorates, hypoglycemia (glucose <70 mg/dL) can be an issue, regardless of whether the patient is diabetic or not. There is a significant risk of death within 1 day of a hypoglycemic episode in all patients, but especially in those with CKD, according to a 2009 study (**Box 7**).[33]

Antiplatelet medication
CKD alone is not a contraindication to antiplatelet therapy. Although nonsteroidal anti-inflammatory drugs (NSAIDs) are contraindicated, aspirin can be safely used in most settings. Other agents, such as clopidogrel or the newer antiplatelet medications, also should be used when indicated.[32]

Glucose control in diabetic patients
In patients with CKD, a target hemoglobin A1c of 7.0% is recommended to prevent the progression of microvascular complications.[12] In a patient in whom recurrent hypoglycemia is a problem, any value lower than 7.0% is not recommended. In those patients with multiple comorbidities and in whom there is a limited life expectancy, this value may be exceeded.[12]

Box 7
Causes of hypoglycemia in CKD

Oral hypoglycemic agents, other medications	Diminished glycogen stores
Delayed degradation of insulin (endogenous or injected) by decreased renal function	
Decreased gluconeogenesis	Deceased oral intake from uremia or gastroparesis
Alcohol	Infection/sepsis
Impaired counterregulatory mechanisms	

Data from Moen MF, Zhan M, Hsu VD, et al. Frequency of hypoglycemia and its significance in chronic kidney disease. Clin J Am Soc Nephrol 2009:4(6):1121–7.

Dietary counseling in chronic kidney disease
All patients with CKD should be evaluated by a dietician skilled in the care of patients with CKD, for comprehensive dietary recommendations. *It is recommended that patients with CKD restrict their sodium to less than 2 g per day or sodium chloride intake to less than 5 g per day.*[12] Excess salt in the diet can not only lead to edema and aggravate hypertension, but will also blunt or negate the effect of diuretics and other antihypertensive medications.

Any patient with CKD should avoid excessive protein (>1.3 gm/kg/day) regardless of their stage.[12] Those patients whose GFR is less than 30 mL/min/1.73 m^2 should decrease their protein intake to 0.8 g/kg/day. If a patient begins to show recurrent nausea, vomiting, auto-protein restriction, and weight loss (all signs of advanced uremia), then the initiation dialysis is indicated. Malnutrition is a powerful predictor of mortality in patients who are on dialysis.

Lipid control
Hyperlipidemia is a frequent complication of proteinuric renal disease (nephrotic syndrome) and diabetes. It also may reflect underlying cardiovascular disease or complicate preexisting disease. As cardiovascular disease is the most common cause of death in patients with CKD, its recognition and treatment are essential.

All patients with CKD should have a full fasting lipid profile drawn, which includes total cholesterol, high-density lipoprotein cholesterol (HDL-C), low-density lipoprotein cholesterol (LDL-C), and triglycerides. If elevated, it should be treated with statin therapy and other lipid-lowering agents, as indicated.[12] There are some conflicting data that suggest that lipid lowering may slow the progression of CKD, perhaps in a similar way as seen in coronary heart disease.[34]

Parathyroid, calcium, phosphorus, and vitamin D
Hyperphosphatemia, from impaired phosphorus excretion, is seen in advanced CKD, and is a stimulus for the secretion of parathyroid hormone (PTH).[35] Hypocalcemia, specifically decreased ionized calcium, further aggravates this elevation. Once the GFR is less than 30 mL/min/1.73 m^2, secondary hyperparathyroidism becomes more clinically significant. The most significant metabolite of vitamin D-1, 25 dihydroxycholecalciferol (D_3), is produced in the renal tissues. D_3 is the principal feedback mechanism to shut off the production of PTH. In CKD, less D_3 is produced, thus eliminating the feedback loop mechanism. Other aggravating causes include increased fibroblast growth factor 23, and diminished expression of vitamin D and calcium sensing receptors in the parathyroid gland.[35] Untreated, the parathyroid gland will hypertrophy, as the demand for more PTH increases unabated (**Box 8, Fig. 4**).[35]

Box 8
Causes of CKD-related hyperparathyroidism

Hyperphosphatemia (from decreased excretion)

Low ionized calcium levels

Low levels of 1,25 dihydroxycholecalciferol (D_3)

Increased fibroblast growth factor 23

Decreased expression of vitamin D and calcium-sensing receptors in the parathyroid gland

Data from Cunningham J, Locatelli F, Rodriguez M. Secondary hyperparathyroidism, disease progression, and therapeutic options. Clin J Am Soc Nephrol 2011;6(4):913.

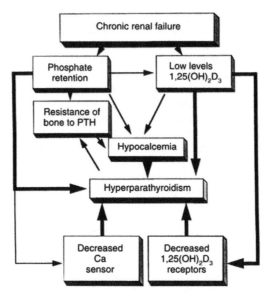

Fig. 4. Chronic renal failure flowchart. (*From* Slatopolsky E, Brown A, Dusso A. Pathogenesis of secondary hyperparathyroidism. Kidney Int 1999;56:S14–9.)

Renal osteodystrophy has numerous manifestations, including osteitis fibrosis cystica, osteomalacia, mixed uremic osteodystrophy, and adynamic bone disease. All of these conditions make the patient much more susceptible to major bone fracture, which can lead to significant morbidity and mortality.

Limiting dietary phosphorus and early referral to a renal dietician can be helpful early in CKD.[35] Later, drugs to bind phosphorus in the gut are used to maintain a normal level. Binders containing aluminum are not recommended, as they can lead to aluminum deposition in the brain and bones. Calcium-based binders also are no longer recommended, as they may lead to coronary calcification in an already high-risk patient.[36]

Elevated PTH levels are treated with vitamin D_3 or one of its analogues, along with a phosphate binder, closely following the PTH level. A new class of drugs, calcimimetics, act on the calcium-sensing receptor of the parathyroid gland. This mechanism, along with D_3 supplementation, may work to more effectively lower the PTH level to near normal.[12]

In addition, patients with CKD should be tested for bone density, but bisphosphonate medication should be avoided in those with a GFR less than 30 mL/min/1.73 m^2.[12]

Anemia and acidosis

Anemia *Normocytic normochromic anemia is a common feature of CKD and is related to decreased production of erythropoietin.*[37] An exception to this is polycystic kidney disease, in which even when patients are on dialysis, their hemoglobin frequently remains normal. *Nonrenal causes of anemia need to be excluded,* including gastrointestinal causes, in the evaluation of patients with CKD and anemia. These include iron deficiency, B12, folate deficiencies, gastrointestinal bleeding, and malignancy.[12]

Anemia is defined as a hemoglobin concentration of less than 13 g/dL in men and 12 g/dL in women. Treatment with erythrocyte stimulating agents, such as erythropoietin or darbepoetin alfa, is indicated when the hemoglobin is less than 10 g/dL.[12] Once treatment has begun, the patient's iron studies, iron, total iron-binding capacity, saturation of transferrin, and ferritin levels need to be closely followed, as significant iron deficiency can develop with therapy.[12]

Acidosis A mild to moderate hyperchloremic (non-anion gap) metabolic acidosis is another common feature in patients with CKD. *Studies have shown that patients with CKD with a serum bicarbonate level less than 22 mg/dL have a higher mortality compared with those whose bicarbonate levels are normal* (**Boxes 9** and **10**).[38]

Treatment with sodium bicarbonate tablets at doses of 650 mg 2 to 3 times a day can slow the decline in CKD, increase strength and nutrition, and inhibit bone-buffering effects of the acidosis. This should be started once the bicarbonate level is less than 22 mg/dL.[39] Dietary counseling with promotion of low acid and higher bicarbonate (or alkaline) food also is helpful.

Cardiovascular Consultation

CKD of any type is a coronary heart disease equivalent and cardiovascular disease is the most common cause of death in this population.[12] Peripheral vascular disease is another common cause of mortality and morbidity. Patients need to be closely evaluated for early signs and symptoms and appropriate referral made to ensure proper evaluations when needed. *CKD should never be a contraindication to diagnostic testing (ie, angiography) or referral, when indicated.*[12]

Avoiding Nephrotoxins

Many medications that are metabolized or excreted by the kidney need to be avoided, discontinued, or the dosages adjusted in the face of CKD.[12] Some of these common medications include nonsteroidal anti-inflammatory medication, sulfa-based medications including antibiotics, cold medication, over-the-counter protein supplements, herbal or "natural products," phosphate-containing bowel preparations or laxatives, antacids or laxatives containing magnesium or aluminum, and salt substitutes, as they contain potassium chloride. Aminoglycosides, normally given in the hospital setting, need to be carefully monitored if given at all. Lithium, digoxin, and calcineurin inhibitors, if necessary, need to be monitored closely with frequent measurement of electrolytes and renal function.[12]

Contrast Studies and MRI

Contrast studies
Patients with CKD are at especially high risk for AKI after contrast infusion; hence, iodinated contrast media given for computed tomography scan, angiography, or

---

Box 9
Causes of metabolic acidosis in CKD

Inability to excrete daily acid load/decreased tubular secretion of hydrogen and organic cations

Decreased ammonium excretion

Decreased bicarbonate regeneration

Accumulation of organic acids, phosphates, and sulfates

Renal tubular acidosis (Type IV most common)

Data from Kraut JA, Kurtz I. Metabolic acidosis of CKD: diagnosis, clinical characteristics, and treatment. Am J Kidney Dis 2005;45:978–93.

Box 10
Consequences of acidosis of CKD

Impaired cardiac function

Impaired oxygen delivery and utilization

Increased secondary hyperparathyroidism and bone damage from buffering

Increased inflammation

Muscle wasting

Increased respiratory effort for compensation

Decreased activity of the Na-K pump

---

venography should be used with caution.[12] A nephrology consultation is helpful in addressing the adequate preparation for these patients. A number of agents and methods have been tried with varying results (**Box 11**).

Nephrotoxic medications NSAIDs, aminoglycosides, diuretics, vancomycin, amphotericin B, cyclosporine, lithium, calcineurin inhibitors.[40]

Acetylcysteine *The role of acetylcysteine in the prevention of contrast-induced nephropathy remains controversial, as a number of studies have had different outcomes.*[41] As it is relatively low cost and low risk, it can be used, but it cannot substitute for adequate hydration. Two 600-mg doses, twice a day the day before, during the procedure, or 1200 mg twice the day of the procedure can be used.
The use of mannitol, loop diuretics, or postprocedure dialysis in patients with advanced CKD not yet on dialysis is not recommended.[40]

Note concerning metformin Although metformin does not cause AKI, it can precipitate a lactic acidosis that can lead to death. Because of this, it should be withheld the day of the procedure and for 48 hours after, while monitoring renal function.[40]
In patients with an Scr greater than 1.5 mg/dL, prophylactic measures need to be undertaken to minimize the risk of contrast-induced nephropathy.[40] Volume expansion can be accomplished with either intravenous normal saline or a sodium bicarbonate mixture of 150 mEq of sodium bicarbonate (3 ampules of 50 mL sodium bicarbonate mixed with 850 mL of sterile water or 5% dextrose). The fluid should be started at a minimum of at least 1 to 2 hours before the procedure at a rate of 1 mL/kg per hour, but preferably this should be started 6 to 12 hours before the procedure and

---

Box 11
High-risk patients for AKI after contrast infusion

CKD	Cardiovascular disease
Diabetes mellitus	Cirrhosis
Acute kidney injury (current)	Nephrotic syndrome
Hypotension/sepsis	Dehydration
Age >70 years	Recent or repeated contrast studies
Myeloma	Intra-arterial > intravenous injection
Organ transplantation	High osmolar contrast
HIV	Volume of contrast

Data from Gupta RK, Bang TJ. Prevention of contrast-induced nephropathy in interventional radiological practice. Semin Intervent Radiol 2010;27:348–59.

continued for 6 to 12 hours after the procedure.[40] *In general, the greater the degree of CKD, the longer the hydration schedule before and after the procedure.*[41]

In summary *Early recognition of CKD, adequate hydration before and after the procedure, acetylcysteine, maintaining adequate blood pressure, minimal volume of preferably nonionic contrast via the intravenous route, and at least 48 hours before another procedure will minimize further damage to the kidney.*

MRI with gadolinium
Nephrogenic systemic fibrosis is a rare condition seen in patients with advanced CKD, a GFR less than 30 mL/min/1.75 m^2, or AKI. A number of studies have implicated the use of gadolinium as a contrast agent for MRI in many of the cases.[42,43] The American College of Radiology has issued a caution in patients whose GFR is between 30 and 44 mL/min/1.75 m^2 or in patients with AKI.[44] If there is no alternative to gadolinium and the patient has a functioning vascular access for hemodialysis (GFR <30 mL/min/ 1.75 m^2), hemodialysis is recommended after the procedure.[45] In a patient with a GFR between 15 and 30 mL/min/1.75 m^2 and no vascular access, hemodialysis is not recommended, because of risk to benefit of gadolinium removal versus temporary access, but consideration should be given to an alternative imaging procedure.[45]

Early Referral to a Nephrologist

In the foregoing discussion, patients with CKD present with marked alterations in their physiology, both from the primary disease processes and from the CKD itself. A number of interventions taken early on in the clinical course can potentially either reverse the damage or slow down its progression. As in many conditions, early recognition is the key factor. A consultant skilled in this can be valuable and sometimes life-saving to the patient (**Box 12, Fig. 5**).

In a patient with CKD, early referral to a nephrologist can establish a partnership with the PCP to treat many of the complications, such as hypertension, anemia, secondary hyperparathyroidism, and acidosis. As part of early referral, dietary counseling about

---

Box 12
Indication for nephrology referral

Acute kidney injury or abrupt decline in GFR

GFR less than 30 mL/min

Persistent albuminuria or proteinuria ACR greater than 300 mg/g or polymerase chain reaction greater than 500 mg/g

Progression of CKD

Urinary RBC casts or RBCs otherwise not explained

CKD and hypertension refractory to 4 or more medications

Structural abnormalities (eg, Polycystic kidney disease (PKD), horseshoe kidney)

Recurrent renal lithiasis

Persistent electrolyte or acid-base disorders

Hereditary kidney disease

Data from Kidney Disease: Improving Global Outcomes (KDIGO) Work Group. KDIGO Clinical practice guidelines for the evaluation and management of chronic kidney disease. Kidney Int Suppl 2013;3:1–150.

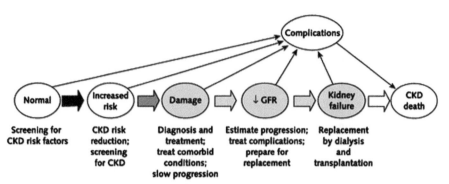

Fig. 5. Progression of chronic kidney disease. (*From* Levey AS, Eckardt KU, Tuskamoto Y. Definition and classification of chronic kidney disease: a position statement from Kidney Disease: Improving Global Outcomes (KDIGO). Kidney Int 2005;67:2092.)

sodium, protein, and phosphorus is part of the *team approach.*[45] For those patients with advanced CKD, education in options for renal replacement therapy (RRT) (ie, hemodialysis vs peritoneal dialysis), timing of the placement of vascular access, insurance issues, and transplantation information create an easier transition for the patients and their caregivers (**Boxes 13–16**).

Good communication and coordinated care between the PCP and consultant will ease the transition to RRT or transplantation.

Preparing for Renal Replacement Therapy

Facing advanced CKD, which may include dialysis or transplantation, can be frightening and intimidating to most patients. A team approach, which includes the PCP, nephrologist, and their team (eg, dietician, social worker, surgeon) can make the transition to RRT for the patient much easier. *It is recommended that a patient be referred at least 1 year before the institution of RRT.*[12] Most nephrologists encourage patients to continue their ongoing relationship with their PCP for a variety of non-CKD–related health care issues. *As important as any intervention in CKD is the role of education of the patients and their family*[12] to assist them in walking through what appears to be a difficult and trying process. In the education process, the nephrology team needs to communicate with the PCP regularly as to the patient's ongoing condition outcome.

Box 13
Benefits of early referral

Treatment and potential reversal of underlying renal dysfunction

Lower mortality and morbidity and better potential for rehabilitation

Shorter hospitalization duration, cost savings

Marked improved survival (both at 3 months and 5 years)

Less need for emergent dialysis and utilization of temporary catheters

Knowledge of medications to limit or avoid

Healthier patients at the start of renal replacement therapy

Data from Huisman RM. The deadly risk of late nephrology referral. Nephrol Dial Transplant 2004;19:2175–80.

Box 14
Consequences of late nephrology referral

Treating complications of uremia
Uncontrolled fluid and electrolyte issues
Anemia
Preventable costs

Malnutrition
Prolonged hospital times
Increased mortality and morbidity
Use of temporary catheters

Data from Wamunno MD, Harris DC. The need for early nephrology referral. Kidney Int Suppl 2005;(94):s128–32.

Box 15
Barriers to early referral

Lack of awareness of CKD

Patient denial or refusal
Other significant comorbidities (eg, cancer, cardiovascular or hepatic conditions)

Health plan stipulations (need for a primary care provider [PCP] referral)
Fear of dialysis, financial fears

Data from Bouware LE, Troll MU, Jaar BG, et al. Identification and referral of patients with progressive CKD: a national study. Am J Kidney Dis 2006;48(2):192–204.

Box 16
PCP referral issues

Lack of available nephrologist (rare in the United States)

Poor relationship between PCP and nephrologists

Fear of losing patients

Lack of awareness of benefits from early referral and current recommendations

Data from Bouware LE, Troll MU, Jaar BG, et al. Identification and referral of patients with progressive CKD: a national study. Am J Kidney Dis 2006;48(2):192–204.

Box 17
Indications to start dialysis

Symptomatic uremia (nausea, anorexia, weight loss, pruritus, myoclonus, cognitive impairment, bleeding, pericarditis, or pleuritis)

Volume overload refractory to diuretics

Electrolyte abnormalities

Acidosis

Deterioration of nutritional status or quality of life

Data from Kidney Disease: Improving Global Outcomes (KDIGO) Work Group. KDIGO clinical practice guidelines for the evaluation and management of chronic kidney disease. Kidney Int Suppl 2013;3:1–150.

Although there is no absolute GFR when RRT is initiated, it is generally started when less than 10 mL/min/1.73 m². Symptoms prompting its start include symptomatic uremia (nausea, anorexia, pruritus, cognitive impairment, myoclonus, bleeding, pericarditis, or pleuritis), refractory volume overload, electrolyte abnormalities, deterioration of nutritional status, and acidosis (**Box 17**).

In some patients, RRT is not indicated or desired by the patients or their families. Nephrology referral can assist in providing assistance and education in the option of conservative, nondialytic management and end-of-life care, again coordinated with the PCP.[12]

REFERENCES

1. Kidney disease statistics for the United States. National Kidney and Urological Disease Information Clearinghouse; U. S. Department of Health and Human Services National Institutes of Health; 2012. p. 1–15 NIH Publication Number 12-3895.
2. Smart NA, Titus TT. Outcomes of early versus late nephrology referral in chronic kidney disease: a systemic review. Am J Med 2011;124(11):1073–80.
3. Wavamunno MD, Harris CH. The need for early nephrology referral. Kidney Int Suppl 2005;67(94):s128–32.
4. Huisman RM. The deadly risk of late referral. Nephrol Dial Transplant 2009;19: 2175–80.
5. Murphy SL, Xu J, Kochanek KD. Deaths: final data for 2010. Natl Vital Stat Rep 2013;61(4):1–117 U. S. Department of Health and Human Services Centers for Disease Control.
6. Baldwin MD, Hariman RJ, Gandhi VC, et al. Management of ischemic heart disease in hemodialysis patients. Semin Dial 1993;6:383–6.
7. Iff S, Craig JC, Turner R, et al. Reduced estimated GFR and cancer mortality. Am J Kidney Dis 2014;63(1):23–30.
8. Bidani AK, Polichowski AJ, Loutzenhiser R, et al. Renal microvascular dysfunction, hypertension and CKD progression. Curr Opin Nephrol Hypertens 2013; 22(1):1–9.
9. Baldwin MD. Assessing cardiovascular risk factors and selecting agents to successfully treat patients with type 2 diabetes mellitus. J Am Osteopath Assoc 2011;111(7 Suppl 5):S2–12.
10. National Kidney Foundation. K/DOQI clinical practice guidelines for chronic kidney disease: evaluation, classification and stratification. Am J Kidney Dis 2002; 39(2 Suppl 1):S1–266.
11. Levey AS, Eckardt KU, Tsukamoto Y, et al. Definition and classification of chronic kidney disease: a position statement from Kidney Disease: Improving Global Outcomes (KDIGO). Kidney Int 2005;67:2089–100.
12. Kidney Disease: Improving Global Outcomes (KDIGO) Work Group. KDIGO Clinical practice guidelines for the evaluation and management of chronic kidney disease. Kidney Int Suppl 2013;3:1–150.
13. Rose BD. Clinical physiology of acid-base and electrolyte disorders. 4th edition. New York: McGraw Hill; 1994. p. 53–4.
14. Levey AS, Coresh J, Greene T, et al. Using standardized serum creatinine values in the modification of diet in renal disease study equation for estimating glomerular filtration rate. Ann Intern Med 2006;145:247–54.
15. Levey AS, Stevens LA, Schmid CH, et al. A new equation to estimate the glomerular filtration rate. Ann Intern Med 2009;150:604–12.

16. Eddy AA. Proteinuria and interstitial injury. Nephrol Dial Transplant 2004;19(2): 277–81.
17. Ginsburg JM, Chang BS, Matarese RA, et al. Use of single voided urine samples to estimate quantitative proteinuria. N Engl J Med 1983;309:1543–6.
18. Cooper R, Rotimi C. Hypertension in blacks. Am J Hypertens 1997;10:804–12.
19. Prather AA, Blumenthal JA, Hinderliter AL, et al. Ethnic differences in the effect of the DASH diet on nocturnal blood pressure dipping in individuals with high blood pressure. Am J Hypertens 2011;24:1338–44.
20. Madhavan SM, O'Toole JF, Konieczkowski M, et al. APOL 1 localization in the normal kidney and non diabetic kidney disease. J Am Soc Nephrol 2011; 22(11):2119–28.
21. Parsa A, Kao WH, Xie D, et al. APOL 1 risk variants, race, and progression of chronic kidney disease. N Engl J Med 2013;369:2183–96.
22. Kriz W, Le Hir M. Pathway to nephron loss starting from glomerular diseases—insights from animal models. Kidney Int 2005;67:404–19.
23. Hostetter TH, Ibraham HN. Aldosterone in chronic kidney and cardiac disease. J Am Soc Nephrol 2003;14:2395–401.
24. Stefanski A, Schmidt KC, Waldherr R, et al. Early increases in blood pressure and diastolic left ventricular function in patients with glomerulonephritis. Kidney Int 1996;50:1321–6.
25. Flack JM, Sica DA, Bakris G, et al. Management of high blood pressure in blacks: an update of the International Society on Hypertension in Blacks Consensus Statement. Hypertension 2010;56:780–800.
26. Chapman N, Dobson J, Wilson S. Effect of spironolactone on blood pressure in subjects with resistant hypertension. Hypertension 2007;49(4):839–45.
27. Hsu TW, Liu JS, Hung SC, et al. Renoprotective effects of renin-angiotensin system blockade in patients with predialysis advanced chronic kidney disease. JAMA Intern Med 2014;174(3):347–54. http://dx.doi.org/10.1001/jamainternmed.2013. 12700.
28. K/DOQI clinical practice guidelines and antihypertensive agents in chronic kidney disease. Available at: http://www.kidney.org/Professionals/kdoqi/guidelines_bp/index.htm. Accessed April 24, 2014.
29. Friedel HA, Buckley MM. Torasemide. A review of its pharmacological properties and therapeutic potential. Drugs 1991;41(1):81–103.
30. Bakris GL, Weir MR, Secic M, et al. Differential effects of calcium antagonist subclasses on markers of nephropathy progression. Kidney Int 2004;65:1991–2002.
31. Navaneethan SD, Nigwekar SU, Sehgal AR, et al. Aldosterone antagonists for preventing the progression of CKD: a systemic review and meta-analysis. Clin J Am Soc Nephrol 2009;4:542–51.
32. Herminda RC. Ambulatory blood pressure monitoring in the prediction of cardiovascular events and effects of chronotherapy: rationale and design of the MAPEC study. Chronobiol Int 2007;24(4):749–75.
33. Moen MF, Zhan M, Hsu VD. Frequency of hypoglycemia and its significance in chronic kidney disease. Clin J Am Soc Nephrol 2009;4(6):1121–7.
34. Fink HA, Ishani A, Taylor BC. Screening for, monitoring, and treatment of chronic kidney disease stages 1 to 3: a systemic review for the U.S. Preventative Service Task Force and for the American College of Physicians Clinical Practice Guideline. Ann Intern Med 2012;156(8):570–81.
35. Cunningham J, Locatelli F, Rodriguez M. Secondary hyperparathyroidism: pathogenesis, disease progression, and therapeutic options. Clin J Am Soc Nephrol 2011;6(4):913–21.

36. Russo D, Miranda J, Ruocco C, et al. The progression of coronary calcifications in predialysis patients on calcium carbonate or sevalamir. Kidney Int 2007;72: 1255–61.
37. Eschback JW. Erythropoietin 1991—an overview. Am J Kidney Dis 1991; 18(4 suppl):3–9.
38. Kovesdy CP, Anderson JE, Kalantar-Zadek K. Association of serum bicarbonate level with mortality in patients with non-dialysis dependent CKD. Nephrol Dial Transplant 2009;24:1232.
39. Kovesdy CP. Pathogenesis, consequences, and treatment of metabolic acidosis in chronic kidney disease. Available at: UpToDate.com. Accessed April 22, 2014.
40. Gupta RK, Bang TJ. Prevention of contrast-induced nephropathy in interventional radiological practice. Semin Intervent Radiol 2010;27:348–59.
41. Nallamothu BK, Shojana KG, Saint S, et al. Is acetylcysteine effective in preventing contrast-related nephropathy? A meta-analysis. Am J Med 2004;20:193–200.
42. Marckmann P, Skov L, Rossen K, et al. Nephrogenic systemic fibrosis: suspected causative role gadodiamide used for contrast-enhanced magnetic resonance imaging. J Am Soc Nephrol 2006;17:2359–62.
43. Sadowski EA, Bennett LK, Chan MR. Nephrogenic systemic fibrosis: risk factors and incidence estimation. Radiology 2007;243:148–57.
44. ACR Committee on Drugs and Contrast Media. ACR manual. American College of Radiology; 2013. p. 81–9, 9.
45. Available at: http://www.uptodate.com/contents/nephrogenic-systemic-fibrosis-nephrogenic-fibrosing-dermopathy-in-advanced-renal-failure. Accessed April 15, 2014.

Evaluation and Management of the Older Adult with Chronic Kidney Disease

Kenya M. Rivas Velasquez, MD, Elizabeth Hames, DO*, Hady Masri, DO

KEYWORDS

- Chronic kidney disease (CKD) • Acute kidney injury (AKI) • Kidney failure
- Renal replacement therapy (RRT) • Older adult

KEY POINTS

- The medical and economic burden of chronic kidney disease (CKD) is borne disproportionally by the geriatric population.
- The older kidney is capable of maintaining homeostasis of body fluids and electrolytes but has limited physiologic reserves.
- Avoidance of nephrotoxic agents is an important aspect of the management of patients with CKD.
- The geriatric population with CKD is at heightened risk for acute kidney injury, which predisposes to worsening CKD.
- Comprehensive geriatric assessment and shared decision making are vital for determining the appropriate management of older adults with CKD.

EPIDEMIOLOGY OF CHRONIC KIDNEY DISEASE

In the United States, 20 million adults have chronic kidney disease (CKD). Less than 2% progress to end-stage renal disease (ESRD), as most patients with CKD will die of a cardiovascular event before then.[1–4] The incidence of CKD in the United States is increasing, most rapidly in people aged 65 years and older. The incidence of recognized CKD in people aged 65 years and older more than doubled between 2000 and 2008.

Department of Geriatrics, Nova Southeastern University College of Osteopathic Medicine, 3200 South University Drive, Ft. Lauderdale, FL 33328, USA
* Corresponding author.
E-mail address: hames@nova.edu

Prim Care Clin Office Pract 41 (2014) 857–874
http://dx.doi.org/10.1016/j.pop.2014.08.006
0095-4543/14/$ – see front matter © 2014 Elsevier Inc. All rights reserved.
primarycare.theclinics.com

The prevalence of CKD in people older than 60 years increased from 19% to 25% in the last decade. The numbers underestimate the reality, as 40% of diabetic patients have unknown stage 1 and 2 CKD. Recent data also reveal that by 65 years of age, almost half of the population will have moderate impairment of kidney function (stage 3 CKD), and around 45% of that will be attributed to diabetes mellitus.[5,6] In addition, acute kidney injury (AKI) continues to be a challenge in all settings of elder care and has implications for CKD. AKI affects 2% to 7% of hospitalized patients, 35% of critically ill patients in the intensive care unit, with a significant amount being in the elderly population. There has been a paradigm shift from the belief that elderly patients with AKI returned back to their premorbid renal states. Rather, studies have shown that AKI may, in turn, cause worsening of preexisting CKD and advance those patients into the more severe stages of CKD.[7-9]

The number of patients older than 65 years with ESRD nearly doubled in the last 25 years.[10] The fastest growing population of patients with ESRD is older than 75 years. More than 44% of the new cases of ESRD are related to diabetes.[11]

DEFINITION OF CHRONIC KIDNEY DISEASE

Accepted as a definition internationally, The National Kidney Foundation Kidney Disease Outcomes Quality Initiative (NKF/DOQI) workgroup defines CKD as the following:

1. The presence of markers of kidney damage for 3 or more months, as defined by structural and functional abnormalities of the kidney, with or without decreased glomerular filtration rate (GFR) or
2. The presence of GFR less than 60 mL/min/1.73 m^2 for 3 or more months with or without other signs of kidney damage[12]

PHYSIOLOGIC CHANGES OF AGING KIDNEY

Kidney function declines after 40 years of age at a mean rate of approximately 1% per year and accelerates slightly in the later years. This finding was reported in a cross-sectional study and confirmed in a population of normal aging persons followed over time. The Baltimore Longitudinal Study demonstrated that two-thirds of a population followed up for 20 years, developed a decline in GFR, whereas the other third remained intact, concluding that age by itself is not necessarily a risk factor for kidney dysfunction.[13]

Renal mass decreases by 25% to 30% between 30 and 80 years of age, with the steepest decline after 50 years. Fat and fibrosis replace some of the remaining functional parenchyma. Loss occurs primarily in the renal cortex and preferentially affects those nephrons most important to maximal urine concentration. Thus, nocturia or frequency with dilute urine is a common finding. Although there is a loss of glomerular mass with aging, the loss of tubular mass is proportional, so that glomerular-tubular balance is usually maintained.

Normal aging is associated with diffuse sclerosis of glomeruli to the extent that 30% of glomeruli are destroyed by 75 years of age. The remaining glomeruli have impaired filtering ability.[14] Intrarenal vascular changes include spiraling of the afferent arterioles, narrowing of the larger arteries, interstitial fibrosis, and shunts between afferent and efferent arterioles allowing blood to bypass the glomeruli.[15] These changes may exacerbate essential hypertension (HTN). At baseline, renal plasma blood flow is 40% lower in healthy normotensive older men than in young men.

On the other hand, older kidneys may be maintained in the state of vasodilation to compensate for loss of vasculature, under the influence of prostaglandins. Vasodilating prostaglandins are increased at baseline in normal older adults, and this contributes to the increased risk of renal injury with the use of nonsteroidal antiinflammatory drugs (NSAIDs) in older people.[16]

Despite significant anatomic and functional changes, the older kidney is still capable of maintaining homeostasis of body fluids and electrolytes under most circumstances. However, under environmental and disease-related stresses, such as volume changes or alterations in acid-base status, the older kidney is slower to respond to correct the abnormality.

In the setting of dehydration, the minimum urine flow rate is twice as great in those older than 70 years compared with those younger than 40 years; the maximum urine osmolality is also reduced with age, reflecting the loss of concentrating ability.[17] The older kidney is more prone to nephrotoxicity related to medications or intravenous (IV) contrast. The injured older kidney is less likely to recover from acute insult.[18] The older kidney is also more vulnerable to ischemic insult, with a greater number of cells undergoing apoptosis following ischemia than in the young kidney.[19] **Table 1** summarizes the anatomic and functional changes of age-related renal changes.

STAGES OF CHRONIC KIDNEY DISEASE

The clinical presentation of kidney disease in older and younger adults is not significantly different. To some extent, CKD is preventable and, if diagnosed early, progression can be halted or slowed and cardiovascular disease prevented.[20] The first hint of kidney disease may be seen on a screening urinalysis demonstrating hematuria, proteinuria, pyuria, and casts in otherwise asymptomatic patients.

The comorbidity associated with the aging process, including vascular disease, diabetes mellitus, and cardiac disease, places older adults at an increased risk for renal insult. As in young adults, diabetes mellitus is the most common cause

Table 1	
Age-related anatomic and functional changes of renal function	
Anatomic	**Functional**
• Decrease in renal mass, mostly from cortex	• Decreased renal blood flow
• Increased renal fat and fibrosis	• Decreased creatinine clearance
• Sclerosis of cortical nephrons with longest loops of Henle	• Impaired sodium excretion and conservation
	• Decreased potassium excretion and conservation
	• Decreased concentrating and diluting capacity
	• Impaired excretion of acid loads
	• Decreased serum rennin and aldosterone
	• Altered intrarenal nitric oxide actions
	• Increased dependence on renal prostaglandins to maintain intrarenal perfusion
	• Decreased vitamin D activation
	• Increased vulnerability to dye, ischemia, or other insults
	• Impaired recovery after insults

Data from Brown WW, Abrass IB, Oreopoulos DG. Introduction: aging and the kidney. Adv Ren Replace Ther 2000;7(1):1–92; and Sands JM. Urine concentrating and diluting ability during aging. J Gerontol A Biol Sci Med Sci 2012;67:1352.

of CKD; diabetic nephropathy is the leading cause of end-stage renal failure, accounting for more than 1 of every 3 patients who enter dialysis or transplantation programs.

Recognizing the various stages of CKD helps the clinician to make informed therapeutic decisions. Staging kidney damage is done by calculating the estimated GFR (eGFR). This measure is the most useful and accepted measure of kidney function.

The creatinine clearance (CrCl) is the most reproducible measure of GFR available. In older adults, creatinine production decreases at nearly the same rate as the renal clearance of creatinine; a normal serum creatinine may actually reflect a decline in kidney function. Based on this, the relationship between serum creatinine and GFR has prompted several investigators to suggest formulas that could properly correct for the confounding variables: age, weight, gender, height, and so forth. Therefore, different formulas to estimate GFR have been proposed by the NKF[20]:

1. Cockcroft-Gault formula
2. Modification of Diet in Renal Disease (MDRD) study equation
3. Chronic Kidney Disease Epidemiology Collaboration (CKD-EPI) creatinine equation developed in 2009
4. CKD-EPI cystatin C and creatinine 2012 equation

These equations can be found in the NKF Web site or downloaded as free applications to be used at the bedside on handheld devices.

Based on the current evidence, the CKD-EPI equation is considered more accurate in stages 1 to 3, and the MDRD is best for stages 4 to 5. The Cockcroft-Gault formula is the most time tested for calculating dosages in clinical settings.

More research is needed in order to support the use of cystatin C as a biomarker for kidney function or the CKD-EPI cystatin and creatinine 2012 equation before they can be accepted as the gold standard equation for GFR.

There are 5 stages for CKD, and they progress from stage 1 (mild) to stage 5 (severe); staging CKD may help the clinician with therapeutic management. In those individuals with early stage CKD, their renal function declines slowly at a variable rate. The first 3 stages progress asymptomatically, and here is when we as primary care physicians play an important role in early recognition and subsequent treatment.

The NKF provides definitions of the 5 stages of CKD,[20] found in **Table 2**.

Table 2 Staging of CKD		
Stage	**Description**	**GFR (mL/min/1.73 m²)**
1	Kidney damage with normal GFR	$\geq$90
2	Kidney damage with mild GFR	89–60
3A	Mild to moderate GFR	59–45
3B	Moderate GFR	45–30
4	Severe GFR	30–15
5	Kidney failure	<15 or dialysis

From National Kidney Foundation/Disease Outcomes Quality Initiative (NKF/DOQI). K/DOQI clinical practice guidelines for CKD: evolution, classification, and stratification. Am J Kidney Dis 2002;39(Suppl 1):S1.

EVALUATION OF CHRONIC KIDNEY DISEASE

The management of CKD includes treatment of reversible causes of renal disease and slowing the progression of renal dysfunction:

Reversible causes
- There is decreased renal perfusion.
- Avoid the administration of nephrotoxic drugs, including aminoglycoside antibiotics, NSAIDs, and radiographic contrast material. Other medications, like cimetidine, trimethoprim, cefoxitin, and flucytosine, will interfere with creatinine secretion without affecting GFR.
- Diagnose urinary tract obstruction, which is considered in patients with unexplained worsening renal function.

Therapy to decrease the rate of progression in patients with CKD is focused on the following:

- Attain the blood pressure goal; in patients with proteinuric disease, reduce proteinuria. High-quality evidence favors the use of an angiotensin-converting enzyme (ACE) inhibitor or angiotensin II receptor blocker (ARB) as first-line treatment in patients with proteinuric CKD because they will not only decrease the blood pressure but they will also slow down the rate of progression of the disease. The blood pressure goal should be 140/90 mm Hg for younger adults. There is strong evidence to support treating hypertensive persons aged 60 years and older to a blood pressure goal of less than 150/90 mm Hg based on the recently released guidelines from the Joint National Committee.[21]
- Restrict protein intake, as it may decrease the progression of kidney dysfunction, yet the optimal level of protein intake is to be determined.
- Manage hyperlipidemia, as there is some evidence that confirms hyperlipidemia may increase the rate of progression of the renal disease.
- Begin smoking cessation, as it increases the risk of developing kidney disease.
- Treatment of chronic metabolic acidosis with supplemental bicarbonate may decrease the progression to ESRD.

RECOGNIZING ACUTE KIDNEY INJURY AS A RISK FACTOR OF CHRONIC KIDNEY DISEASE

In addition to smoking, medications, HTN, and diabetes, AKI is also a major risk factor for developing CKD and/or worsening stages of CKD. Therefore, it is important to recognize AKI during its early stages and prevent progression. The differential diagnosis and workup of AKI is summarized in **Fig. 1**. The Acute Kidney Injury Network's (AKIN) criteria and the RIFLE (risk, injury, failure, loss, ESRD) criteria (a systematic framework for the definition and stratification of AKI) are similar, both being championed as valid by The Kidney Disease Improving Global Outcomes' (KDIGO) guidelines in 2012.[22,23] RIFLE is an acronym for grading the severity of kidney injury in AKI from *risk* (R), to *injury* (I), to *failure* (F), to the outcomes of *loss* (L) and *ESRD* (E). RIFLE-L (*loss*) is an outcome defined as persistent acute renal failure with a complete loss of renal function for greater than 4 weeks. Finally, RIFLE-E (ESRD) demonstrates that those with AKI may have a poor outcome and require renal replacement therapy (RRT) for 3 months or greater. The AKIN's criteria may capture AKI earlier, as a small increase of 0.3 mg/dL in baseline serum creatinine within a 48-hour period qualifies as stage I AKI. Both the AKIN and RIFLE criteria use serum creatinine and urine output as biomarkers. **Fig. 2** summarizes the various stages of the RIFLE and AKIN criteria when defining AKI.

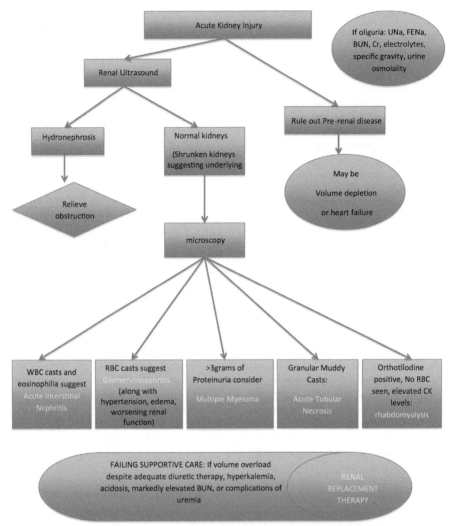

Fig. 1. Differential diagnosis and diagnostic algorithm for AKI. BUN, blood urea nitrogen; CK, creatine kinase; Cr, creatine; RBC, red blood cell; WBC, white blood cell. (*Data from* KDIGO clinical practice guideline for acute kidney injury. Kidney Int Suppl 2012;2(1):1–138.)

EARLIER DETECTION OF ACUTE KIDNEY INJURY: NOVEL BIOMARKERS

Serum creatinine, as a marker of kidney function, has limitations in the sarcopenic elderly population, as it is heavily influenced by muscle mass. In addition, an increase in creatinine may be delayed and not reflect real-time AKI. Newer biomarkers may mitigate this problem. Cystatin C, kidney injury molecule-1, and neutrophil gelatinase–associated lipocalin have been studied and might have utility as early markers in AKI. Although cystatin C may potentially be used in the CKD setting as a more accurate measure of GFR, it may also have a role in the early detection of AKI. Cystatin C also has been reported to increase about 1 to 2 days earlier than serum creatinine in patients developing AKI.[24] With these real-time novel biomarkers, earlier detection of AKI implies earlier intervention, which may curb CKD progression.[25]

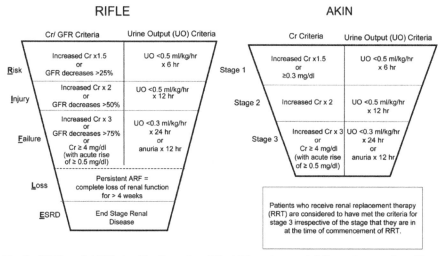

Fig. 2. RIFLE and AKIN classifications for AKI. ARF, acute renal failure; Cr, creatine. (*From* Cruz DN, Ricci Z, Ronco C. Clinical review: RIFLE and AKIN – time for reappraisal. Crit Care 2009;13:211.)

PROGNOSIS OF ACUTE KIDNEY INJURY AND ITS IMPLICATIONS WITH CHRONIC KIDNEY DISEASE

There has been a paradigm shift from the belief that those with AKI return back to their premorbid level of renal function. Several studies show that older patients with AKI may then develop CKD, progression of previously established CKD, or ESRD.[7–9] One study by Ishani and colleagues[7] in 2009, with a mean age of 79.2 years, examined the long-term risk for ESRD among the elderly. Medicare beneficiaries were categorized as having AKI, CKD, both CKD and AKI, or neither condition. On hospital discharge, the incidence of ESRD was examined over a 2-year period. The cohort with both CKD and AKI had the highest hazard ratio for the development of ESRD. In addition, those with AKI and CKD had higher 2-year mortality than those with AKI alone.

Lo and colleagues[8] examined long-term outcomes for those with AKI that required renal in-hospital replacement therapy for further progression of CKD. With a mean age of 63.5 years within this cohort, this 8-year study found that AKI requiring dialysis was associated with a 28- fold increase in developing CKD stage 4, 5, or ESRD.[8]

Using the universal health care system in the Canadian province of Ontario, Wald and colleagues[9] conducted a population-based cohort study that spanned a 10-year period (median follow-up 3 years) on the long-term risk of ESRD and death among hospitalized patients who sustained AKI requiring acute dialysis. With a mean age of 62 years, survivors hospitalized with AKI were approximately 3 more times likely to require chronic dialysis compared with those without AKI.

THE IMPORTANCE OF PREVENTING ACUTE KIDNEY INJURY

Although AKI is a risk factor for developing CKD, CKD is also an identifiable risk factor for developing AKI, which implies a bidirectional relationship between these two conditions. Thus, it is imperative for clinicians to identify at-risk elders prone to AKI. The identifiable risk factors include for AKI include the following:

- Age greater than 75 years
- Hypovolemic states

- CKD
- Heart failure and cardiorenal syndrome
- Liver failure and hepatorenal syndrome
- Diabetes
- Certain medications use
  - NSAIDs
  - Diuretics
  - ACE inhibitors and ARBs
  - Antibiotics such as
    - Trimethoprim-sulfamethoxazole
    - Aminoglycosides
    - Vancomycin
- Radio-contrast studies
- Cardiac bypass surgery

The Kidney Disease Improving Global Outcomes' (KDIGO) guidelines suggest neph-rotoxic agents be discontinued when possible and that good volume status and perfusion pressure should be ensured. In septic patients, long-standing ACE inhibitors and ARB medication may be held. Hyperglycemia may cause excessive diuresis and worsens volume depletion and should be treated aggressively. KDIGO's guidelines suggest keeping blood sugars between 100 and 149 mg/dL in critically ill patients with AKI (2C recommendation). Medication adjustment should be implemented in AKI.[26]

Iodine-based contrast procedures, such as cardiac catheterization and radio imaging, may place these patients at risk for the development of contrast-induced nephropathy (CIN). High-risk patients should be identified; medications, such as NSAIDs, should be held before the procedure. Volume expansion using mainly isotonic (0.9%) saline may helpful in preventing CIN. A study by Trivedi and colleagues[27] of 53 patients undergoing cardiac catheterizations showed the use of IV isotonic saline solution was more effective than encouraging oral fluids in the prevention of CIN-AKI. The use of oral N-acetyl cysteine as well as IV isotonic saline is a 2D recommendation from the KDIGO's 2012 guidelines. Most importantly, one should find alternative, lower-risk radiologic modalities for these high-risk patients when possible.

MANAGEMENT OF DIABETIC NEPHROPATHY IN THE LONG-TERM CARE SETTING

The optimal treatment strategy for long-term care (LTC) patients with diabetic nephropathy is uncertain. Current guidelines have been formulated for community-dwelling persons with diabetic nephropathy. In general, in older adults with functional and cognitive decline associated with limited life expectancy, therapy and glycemic goals should be individualized and relaxed and quality of life prioritized.[28]

The guidelines in LTC patients with diabetic nephropathy who have good functional status and good prognosis include the following:

1. If patients' creatinine levels are increasing or if GFR is declining, consider a protein-restricted diet. It may delay the onset of ESRD in patients with late-stage renal insufficiency.
2. If the albumin/creatinine ratio is less than 30 mcg/mg, yearly evaluation is recommended. Management of diabetes and HTN is advised. Prescribe ACE inhibitors or ARBs if proteinuria or HTN is present of if proteinuria progresses. Consider the use of ACE inhibitors or ARBs even in the absence of HTN. Because ACE inhibitors and

ARBs have protective effects on the kidneys, their use should be considered in all patients who have both type 2 diabetes and HTN. Evidence supports the use of ACE inhibitors in normotensive patients with type 1 diabetes and in normotensive patients with type 2 diabetes.

3. If albumin/creatinine is greater than 300 mcg/mg, recheck in 6 months.[4] (This ratio could be influenced by inflammation, fever, heart failure, uncontrolled HTN, and diabetes.)
4. A nephrologist may be consulted in the following situations if appropriate in the patients' circumstances:
   - Rapid increase in creatinine
   - GFR less than 30 mL/min/1.73 m²
   - Severe HTN
   - Hyperkalemia
   - Cause of nephropathy is unclear

When evaluating DM, in the setting of moderate to severe anemia, a Hemoglobin A1C may not be a reliable diagnostic measure to reflect true glycemic control. Consequently, a fasting glucose or 2-hour postload plasma glucose levels should be considered as a bedside laboratory measurement.[29]

MANAGEMENT OF KIDNEY FAILURE IN OLDER ADULTS
Definitions

Kidney failure and ESRD are commonly confused terms that have 2 distinct definitions. Kidney failure is defined as a level of GFR less than 15 mL/min, with or without signs and symptoms of uremia. ESRD is kidney failure treated with either dialysis or transplantation and is an operational classification not based on the level of kidney function. **Table 3** is a classification of kidney failure, revised by the NKF/DOQI.[30]

CKD can progress to kidney failure in older adults, although kidney failure is less common than earlier stages of CKD in this population. The clinician tending to these patients faces complex medical decision making. Care of the older adult with kidney failure includes comprehensive geriatric assessment, timely referral to a nephrologist, and shared decision-making conversations with patients and caregivers. A framework of validated prognostication tools is available to help guide appropriate intensity of management and is reviewed.

Epidemiology of End-Stage Renal Disease in the United States

The US population older than 65 years is projected to reach more than 70 million by 2030 and more than 80 million by 2050, which is depicted in **Fig. 3**.[31,32]

Table 3	
Revised NKF/DOQI classification of kidney failure	
Stage (based on GFR)	**GFR (mL/min/1.73 m²)**
G5	<15
G5D	<15 and treated with dialysis
Stage (based on albuminuria)	**Urine albuminuria/creatinine ratio**
A3	>300 mg/g

Data from National Kidney Foundation/Disease Outcomes Quality Initiative (NKF/DOQI). K/DOQI clinical practice guidelines for CKD: evolution, classification, and stratification. Am J Kidney Dis 2002;39(Suppl 1):S1.

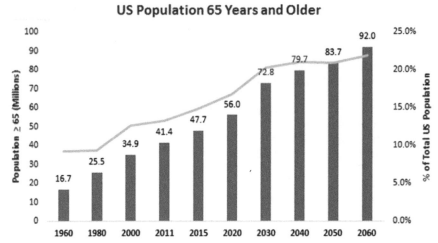

Fig. 3. Projected US population aged 65 years and older. (*From* US Census Bureau. Current population reports. Available at: www.census.gov/prod/1/pop/p25-952.pdf. Accessed on March 2014.)

ESRD is less common among older adults than earlier stages of CKD; however, the number of patients older than 65 years with ESRD nearly doubled in the last 25 years.[10] Among older adults, the fastest growing population of patients with ESRD is older than 75 years.[11] Forty-four percent of new patients with ESRD aged 75 years or older have diabetes.[5] With an aging population and a high incidence of diabetes, there are growing economic implications, such as the current an annual Medicare cost of $87,945 per patient-year for hemodialysis alone.[10]

Risk Factors for Kidney Failure and Disease Progression

In older adults with CKD, there is a greater risk of cardiovascular complications and mortality than of progression to ESRD. Several factors have been shown to significantly increase the risk of kidney failure in older adults[2]:

- Proteinuria
- HTN
- Diabetes
- Race (African American)
- Sex (male)

A major independent risk factor for mortality and the progression of CKD to ESRD is high albuminuria (>300 mg/g of creatinine). This biomarker needs to be monitored frequently and controlled through medical therapy at earlier stages of CKD.[30]

The timing of referral to a nephrologist can have a significant impact on management. For various reasons, patients are sometimes referred late. Late referrals are those that are close in time to the need for RRT, and these are at risk for increased complications and mortality. Shared decision-making conversations addressing initiation or withholding of dialysis for older adults are recommended by the Renal Physicians Association/American Society of Nephrology's guidelines (2010).[33] Data from

Smart and Titus[3] in 2011 showed that early referral to a nephrologist is associated with the following benefits:

- Improved survival
- Informed selection of dialysis type
- Timely placement of access
- Nonemergent dialysis initiation
- Lower morbidity and better rehabilitation
- Fewer and shorter hospital stays
- Lower overall cost of treatment
- Timely transplant when indicated

Approaches to Management of Kidney Failure in Older Adults

Two generalized approaches to the management of older adults with kidney failure are RRT (which includes hemodialysis) and *medical management*.[34] RRT is considered to be a disease-oriented, goal-oriented model. The overall length of patient survival is the most important outcome. Medical management focuses on patient preferences, quality of life, symptom management, and shared decision-making conversations between clinician, patients, and caregivers. There is a current trend favoring medical management in older adults, particularly those with significant frailty and functional decline. Management trends including timing of dialysis initiation, prognostication tools, and appropriate patient selection for hemodialysis are explored in this section.

Renal replacement therapy (disease-oriented model)
Early initiation There is an increasing trend toward earlier initiation of hemodialysis in older adults at higher GFR. Data from Kurella Tamura and colleagues[35] in 2010 identified volume overload, cognitive decline, increased activities-of-daily-living (ADL) dependence, and weight loss as the driving factors for early initiation. However, these factors only accounted for 31% of early dialysis initiation. Other driving factors may include metabolic abnormalities, regional and economic factors, and physician practice style.[33] Early dialysis initiation among older adults has not been shown to improve clinical outcomes or quality of life. The IDEAL (Initiating Dialysis Early and Late) trial of 2010 (N = 828, median age of 60 years) showed no difference in survival or quality of life among patients who started dialysis with a lower GFR (5–7 mL/min) as compared with a GFR of 10 to 14 mL/min, an average of 6 months later in the progression of kidney failure. There was no difference in secondary outcomes of cardiovascular events, infection, or hemodialysis complications.[36]

Quality-of-life implications following dialysis initiation Among nursing home patients, there is a significant and sustained functional decline of dialysis patients. There is a sharp decline of ADL score at the time of dialysis initiation. In a study of 3702 nursing home patients, 58% died and only 13% maintained predialysis function at 1 year after dialysis initiation.[37] Lower physical activity predicts higher 1-year mortality in elderly hemodialysis patients.[38] There is an increasing amount of early withdrawal from hemodialysis among older adults. Up to 30% of patients with ESRD who are older than 75 years withdraw for treatment, suggesting poor tolerance of the procedure and lowered quality of life.[39]

United States regional variation of intensity of end-stage renal disease treatment There is significant regional variation in health care intensity in the last year of life among patients across the United States. These geographic patterns can be seen in terms of Medicare spending for hospitalizations late in life, intensive care use in the last month of life, use of feeding tubes, and overall cost of end-of-life care. Patterns of high-intensity ESRD treatment, represented as lack of discontinuation of dialysis before death, paralleled patterns of high-intensity end-of-life treatment. These high-intensity regions are clustered along the east and west coasts and in southern states. Demographics, patient preferences, physician practice styles, and severity of illness all influence this pattern of care intensity.[40] Older adult patients with kidney failure in these high-spending, high-intensity-of-care regions would be assumed to be better prepared for the initiation of dialysis. However, individuals in high-intensity regions are less likely to be under the care of a nephrologist before ESRD, less likely to have a fistula placed before dialysis initiation, more likely to die in the hospital, and did not self-report improved quality of life.[41]

Medical management (patient-centered model)

Medical management is defined as a patient-centered, individualized care plan. There is more of a focus on quality of life and patient preferences. Symptom management is one of the primary goals. This approach recognizes the complex medical comorbidities and geriatric syndromes (eg, frailty, cognitive decline) of older adults. Signs and symptoms are viewed as overlapping and are not strictly attributed to renal pathophysiology. Disease-specific treatment goals (eg, balancing electrolytes) can still be incorporated into the treatment plan.

Recent guidelines from the NKF/DOQI recommend withholding dialysis in the setting of certain grave medical illnesses conferring limited life expectancy and when dialysis is not tolerated. The guideline does not address other medical comorbidities, functional status, geriatric syndromes (eg, frailty, cognitive decline), or age-specific recommendations. **Box 1** summarizes the recommendations by the NKF/DOQI for withholding dialysis.

The revised Renal Physicians Association/American Society of Nephrology (RPA/ASN) Shared Decision-Making Guideline was recently incorporated into the RPA Clinical Practice Guidelines. This guideline stresses the importance of conversations of shared decision making between physician, patients, and caregivers. It recommends against the initiation of chronic hemodialysis without a comprehensive patient assessment of overall prognosis. The following list highlights some key points of the RPA/ASN Shared Decision-Making Guideline[33]:

- Fully informing patient and caregivers about diagnosis, prognosis, and treatment options
- Institution of advanced care planning
- Consideration of foregoing dialysis if overall prognosis is poor
- Offer palliative care to all patients with kidney failure

Box 1
NKF/DOQI's recommendation for withholding of dialysis

1. Irreversible neurologic dysfunction

2. End-stage cancer

3. Intolerance of the procedure

Data from National Kidney Foundation/Disease Outcomes Quality Initiative (NKF/DOQI). K/DOQI clinical practice guidelines for CKD: evolution, classification, and stratification. Am J Kidney Dis 2002;39(Suppl 1):S1.

A novel strategy of medical management is termed *maximum conservative management*. This strategy is a multidisciplinary supportive approach to care for patients with kidney failure who choose to forego dialysis. This approach is also referred to as *nondialysis treatment*, *palliative renal care*, and *conservative management*. Older adults are offered therapy primarily for symptom management, and hospice or palliative care is implemented based on patient preference. Conditions such as anemia and hyperlipidemia are treated; dietary restrictions are liberal and are tied to symptom management and quality of life. Patients receiving maximum conservative management self-reported better quality of life as compared with those receiving hemodialysis, and overall survival time included fewer hospital days.[42,43] **Table 4** summarizes the treatment strategies and measured outcomes of patients receiving maximum conservative management.

Special Treatment Considerations for Patients with Kidney Failure

Choosing Wisely Campaign
The Choosing Wisely Campaign is an initiative of the American Board of Internal Medicine (ABIM) to promote the effective use of health care resources and can be accessed at www.choosingwisely.org. Recommendation lists have been developed by the ABIM and medical specialty societies. A guideline list from the ABIM, in conjunction with the ASN, includes 3 recommendations for patients categorized as having or approaching kidney failure[44]:

- *DO NOT* perform routine cancer screenings on dialysis patients with limited life expectancy.
- *DO NOT* place peripherally inserted central catheter lines in patients with stage III to V CKD without first consulting a nephrologist (preserve venous sites).
- *DO NOT* initiate chronic dialysis without implementing a shared decision-making process consisting of patients and the physician.

Prognostic Tools for Shared Decision Making in Older Adults
Older adults with multiple comorbidities and geriatric syndromes may not be appropriate candidates for hemodialysis. There is a growing set of validated prognostication tools to aid in the appropriate selection of older adults for RRT. These tools emphasize the importance of assessing patients' overall functional status in the setting of geriatric syndromes. Physician-patient communication is integral to the process through the use of shared decision-making conversations. Several recent prognostication tools are reviewed next.

Table 4	
Maximum conservative management for older adults	
Treatment Strategies	**Measured Outcomes**
Loop diuretics for fluid overload	Fewer hospital days
Only K+ restricted in diet	More likely to die at home
Hemoglobin optimized with Epo/Fe	More likely to die in a hospice
Lipid-lowering medications	Better self-reported quality of life
Calcium and phosphorus balanced	
Hospice/palliative care offered	

Abbreviations: Epo, epoetin; Fe, iron; K, potassium.
Data from Carson RC. Is maximum conservative management an equivalent treatment option to dialysis for elderly patients with significant comorbid disease? Clin J Am Soc Nephrol 2009;(4):1611–9; and Treit K, et al. Timing of dialysis initiation in the geriatric population: toward a patient-centered approach. Semin Dial 2013;26(6):682–9.

Multidimensional Prognostic Index
Comprehensive geriatric assessment of functional status, cognitive abilities, nutritional status, number and severity of medical comorbidities, and medication burden was used to calculate a mortality risk score.

Multidimensional Prognostic Index
- Scoring based on comprehensive geriatric assessment
  - ADLs, instrumental ADLs; Cumulative Illness Rating Scale: number and severity of medical comorbidities; Geriatric Depression Scale; Short Portable Mental Status Questionnaire: 10-question evaluation of cognitive function; Mini-Nutritional Assessment; Exton Smith Scale: risk of pressure ulcers; and medication burden
- Scored as low, moderate, or severe risk of mortality

The Multidimensional Prognostic Index is a significantly more accurate predictor of 1-year mortality for elderly, hospitalized patients with CKD than is a measure of GFR alone.[45]

Department of Veterans Affairs (VA) risk score (2013)
The Department of Veterans Affairs (VA) risk score is a risk-stratification and planning tool to aid in the appropriate selection, preparation, and transitioning of patients to dialysis. It predicts the 1-year risk of progression to ESRD for older adults. A total of 1866 patients aged 65 years and older with a GFR less than 30 were followed at an outpatient VA medical center. Data showed the significant independent risk factors for ESRD were age, low eGFR, low potassium, high systolic blood pressure and heart failure, and low albumin.[46]

Hemodialysis mortality predictor: integrated prognostic model
This validated tool predicts early (6-month) mortality of dialysis (and potential) dialysis patients and can be used to aid in the selection of appropriate candidates. Patients are scored from 0 to 5, with a score of 5 conferring greater than 85% mortality. The Charlson Comorbidity Index was used to measure the number and severity of conditions relative to age. A previously validated surprise question for physicians was incorporated into the assessment: Would I be surprised if this patient died within the next 6 months? Five variables were found to be independently associated with early mortality[47]:

1. Older age
2. Peripheral vascular disease
3. Answer NO to the surprise question to physicians: Would I be surprised if this patient died within the next 6 months?
4. Dementia
5. Low albumin

This mortality predictor tool is currently available free of charge as an online interactive calculator and provides both a percentage and scaled score.

Considerations for starting frail patients on dialysis
Swidler[48] discusses the dilemma of appropriate selection of geriatric patients for RRT. Three phenotypes of dialysis candidates are defined as follows:

- Healthy (optimal) candidates
- Vulnerable patients who had unpredictable outcomes
- Frail patients (often nursing home patients) with frequent poor outcomes

---

Box 2
The frail phenotype

Karnofsky score less than 50 (disabled)

Older age (>85 years)

Geriatric syndromes (dementia, + frailty testing, albumin <35)

Answer *no* to surprise question: Would I be surprised if this patient died in the next 6 months?

Low survival probability (Charlson comorbidity score >8 nursing home patient, hemodialysis mortality predictor)

Data from Swidler M. Considerations in starting a patient with advanced frailty on dialysis: complex biology meets challenging ethics. Clin J Am Soc Nephrol 2013;8:1421–8.

Swidler[48] developed a *frail phenotype* of older adults with significant functional deficits who should forgo dialysis (summarized in **Box 2**). When characterizing the frail phenotype, a comprehensive, multidisciplinary assessment was stressed, including geriatric susceptibility factors, such as frailty, dementia, and function.[46] Medical comorbidities were also considered, using the Charlson comorbidity score and hemodialysis mortality predictor (see the aforementioned number 3). This phenotype was created with an integrated approach, combining geriatric risk factors, medical comorbidities, and survival data.[48]

When assessing and implementing the appropriate management of kidney failure in older adults, comprehensive geriatric assessment and shared decision making is the best option for individualized, patient-centered care.

SUMMARY

The prevalence of CKD in people older than 60 years increased from 19% to 25% in the last decade. The numbers underestimate the reality, as 40% of diabetic patients have unknown stage 1 and 2 CKD and around 45% of that will be attributed to diabetes mellitus. Clinical presentation of kidney disease in older and younger adults is not significantly different. To some extent, CKD is preventable; if diagnosed early, progression can be halted and cardiovascular disease prevented.

The CrCl is the most reproducible measure of GFR available. In older adults, creatinine production decreases at nearly the same rate as the renal clearance of creatinine; a normal serum creatinine may actually reflect a decline in kidney function. This relationship between serum creatinine and GFR has prompted several investigators to suggest formulas that could properly correct for confounding variables, such as age, weight, sex, gender, height, and so forth. Therefore, different formulas to estimate GFR have been proposed by the NKF; they are available in the NKF Web site or downloaded as free applications to be used at the bedside.

It is also important to note the special bidirectional relationship between AKI and CKD. Although CKD is a major risk factor for AKI, AKI is also an identifiable risk factor for CKD. In an effort to curb CKD onset and/or worsening stages of CKD, it is imperative to identify high-risk elderly patients. In addition, it is vital to prevent AKI through avoidance of nephrotoxins, maintenance of adequate volume status, and judicious use of contrast-based radiologic procedures.

The number of older adults with kidney failure is growing rapidly. End-stage kidney disease can be treated with RRT (dialysis or transplantation) or managed medically (conservatively or palliatively). The management of kidney failure in older adults requires comprehensive geriatric assessment, which incorporates detailed functional assessment. There are multiple validated prognostication tools available to assist physicians in the appropriate selection of older adults as hemodialysis candidates. Shared decision-making conversations are recommended for physicians, patients, and caregivers. In older adults with functional and cognitive decline associated with limited life expectancy, management should be individualized, with an emphasis on patient preferences and overall quality of life.

REFERENCES

1. Kidney statistics for the US. National Kidney and Urologic Disease Clearinghouse. Available at: http://kidney.niddk.nih.gov/kudiseases/pubs/kustats/KU_Diseases_Stats_50. Accessed November 15, 2013.
2. Anderson S. Prediction, progression, and outcomes of chronic kidney disease in older adults. J Am Soc Nephrol 2009;20:1199–209.
3. Smart N, Titus T. Outcomes of early versus late nephrology referral in chronic kidney disease: a systematic review. Am J Med 2011;124:10–3.
4. Cooper M. Pathogenesis, prevention, and treatment of diabetic nephropathy. Lancet 1998;352:213–9.
5. Fox CS, Larson MG, Leip EP. Predictors of new-onset kidney disease in a community-based population. JAMA 2004;291:844.
6. de Mendonça A, Vincent JL, Suter PM. Acute renal failure in the ICU: risk factors and outcome evaluated by the SOFA score. Intensive Care Med 2000;26:915–21.
7. Ishani A, Xue JL, Himmelfarb J. Acute kidney injury increases risk of ESRD among elderly. J Am Soc Nephrol 2009;20:223–8.
8. Lo JL, Go AS, Chertow GM. Dialysis-requiring acute renal failure increases the risk of progressive chronic kidney disease. Kidney Int 2009;76:893–9.
9. Wald R, Quinn RR, Luo J. Chronic dialysis and death among survivors of acute kidney injury requiring dialysis. JAMA 2009;302:1179–85.
10. US Renal Data System. 2013 annual data report: atlas of chronic kidney disease and ESRD in the United States. National Institutes of Health; 2013.
11. Rosner M. Geriatric nephrology: responding to a growing challenge. Clin J Am Soc Nephrol 2010;5(5):936–42, 7.
12. Levey AS, Eckardt KV, Tsukamoto Y. Definition and classification of chronic kidney disease: a position statement from kidney disease: improving global outcomes (KDIGO). Kidney Int 2005;67:2089.
13. Brown WW, Abrass IB, Oreopoulos DG. Introduction: aging and the kidney. Adv Ren Replace Ther 2000;7(1):1–92.
14. Nyengaard JR, Bendtsen TF. Glomerular number and size in relation to age, kidney weight, and body surface in normal man. Anat Rec 1992;232:194.
15. Long DA, Mu W, Price KL. Blood vessels and the aging kidney. Nephron Exp Nephrol 2005;101:e95.
16. Field TS, Gurwitz JH, Glynn RJ. The renal effects of non-steroidal anti-inflammatory drugs in older people: findings from the established populations for epidemiologic studies of the elderly. J Am Geriatr Soc 1999;47:507.
17. Sands JM. Urine concentrating and diluting ability during aging. J Gerontol A Biol Sci Med Sci 2012;67:1352.
18. Pucelikova T, Dangas G, Mehran R. Contrast-induced nephropathy. Catheter Cardiovasc Interv 2008;71:62.
19. Schmith R, Cartley LG. The impact of aging on kidney repair. Am J Physiol Renal Physiol 2008;294:F1265–72.

20. Shahady E. Diabetes and Chronic Kidney Disease: Prevention, Early Recognition, and Treatment. Consultant 2014;54(1):20–5.
21. James PA. 2014 evidence-based guideline for the management of high blood pressure in adults. Report from the panel members appointed to the Eight Joint National Committee (JNC8). JAMA 2014;311(5):507–20.
22. Bellomo R, Ronco C, Kellum JA. Acute renal failure - definition, outcome measures, animal models, fluid therapy and information technology needs: the Second International Consensus Conference of the Acute Dialysis Quality Initiative (ADQI) Group. Crit Care 2004;8(4):R204–12.
23. Mehta RL, Kellum JA, Shah SV. Acute kidney injury network: report of an initiative to improve outcomes in acute kidney injury. Crit Care 2007;11(2):R31.
24. Zhang Z, Lu B, Sheng X. Cystatin C in prediction of acute kidney injury: a systemic review and meta-analysis. Am J Kidney Dis 2011;9(3):356–65.
25. Lerma EV, Batuman V. Novel biomarkers of renal function. Medscape 2012.
26. Kidney International. KDIGO clinical practice guideline for acute kidney injury. Kidney Int Suppl 2012;2(1):1–138.
27. Trivedi HS, Moore H, Nasr S. A randomized prospective trial to assess the role of saline hydration on the development of contrast nephrotoxicity. Nephron Clin Pract 2003;93:C29–34.
28. American Diabetes Association. Executive summary: standards of medical care in diabetes. 2014. Diabetes Care 2014;31:S5–11.
29. Starkman HS, Wacks M, Soeldner JS, et al. Effect of acute blood loss on glycosylated hemoglobin determinations in normal subjects. Diabetes Care 1983;6:291–4.
30. National Kidney Foundation/Disease Outcomes Quality Initiative (NKF/DOQI). K/DOQI clinical practice guidelines for CKD: evolution, classification, and Stratification. Am J Kidney Dis 2002;39(Suppl 1):S1.
31. US Census Bureau. Current population reports. Available at: www.census.gov/prod/1/pop/p25-952.pdf. Accessed on March 2014.
32. US Census Bureau. 2008 national population projections. Available at: https://census.gov/population/projections. Accessed on March 2014.
33. Shared decision making in the appropriate initiation of and withdrawal from dialysis. 2nd edition. Renal Physicians Association/American Society of Nephrology; Clinical Practice Guideline, Rockville (MD); 2010.
34. Bowling CB, O'Hare AM. Managing older adults with chronic kidney disease: individualized versus disease-based approaches. Am J Kidney Dis 2012;59(2):293–302.
35. Kurella Tamura M. Signs and symptoms associated with earlier dialysis initiation in nursing home residents. Am J Kidney Dis 2010;56(6):1117–26.
36. Cooper B. A randomized, controlled trial of early versus late initiation of dialysis. N Engl J Med 2009;363(16):1539–47.
37. Kurella Tamura M. Functional status of elderly adults before and after initiation of dialysis. N Engl J Med 2009;361(16):1539–47.
38. Shiplak MG. The presence of frailty in elderly persons with chronic renal insufficiency. Am J Kidney Dis 2004;43:861–7.
39. Muthalagappan S. Dialysis or conservative care for frail older patients: ethics of shared decision making. Nephrol Dial Transplant 2013;28:2717–22.
40. Gessert CE. Regional variation in care at the end of life: discontinuation of dialysis. BMC Geriatr 2013;13:39.
41. O'Hare AM. Regional variation in health care intensity and treatment practices for end-stage renal disease in older adults. JAMA 2010;304(2):180–6.

42. Carson RC. Is maximum conservative management an equivalent treatment option to dialysis for elderly patients with significant comorbid disease? Clin J Am Soc Nephrol 2009;4:1611–9.

43. Treit K. Timing of dialysis initiation in the geriatric population: toward a patient-centered approach. Semin Dial 2013;26(6):682–9.

44. Choosing Wisely Campaign. American Board of Internal Medicine Foundation and American Society of Nephrology Quality and Patient Safety Task Force. 2013. Available at: www.choosingwisely.org. Accessed March 1, 2014.

45. Pilotto A. A multidimensional approach to the geriatric patient with chronic kidney disease. J Nephrol 2010;23(S15):S5–10.

46. Drawz PE. A simple tool to predict end-stage renal disease within 1 year in elderly adults with advanced chronic kidney disease. J Am Geriatr Soc 2013;61:762–8.

47. Cohen LM. Predicting six-month mortality for patients who are on maintenance hemodialysis. Clin J Am Soc Nephrol 2010;5(1):72–9.

48. Swidler M. Considerations in starting a patient with advanced frailty on dialysis: complex biology meets challenging ethics. Clin J Am Soc Nephrol 2013;8:1421–8.

Obesity-related Kidney Disease

Samuel Snyder, DO[a],*, Gracie A. Turner, DO[b], Alan Turner, DO[c]

KEYWORDS

- Obesity • Kidney • Hypertension • Insulin resistance • Inflammation

KEY POINTS

- The prevalence of chronic kidney disease (CKD) is increasing, and the epidemic of obesity is one of the causes.
- Obesity exacerbates hypertension as a risk factor for CKD, activating the renin-angiotensin and sympathetic nervous systems at the level of the adipocyte, causing vasoconstriction and salt and water retention.
- Obesity exacerbates glucose intolerance and insulin resistance as risk factors for CKD, with deposition of abnormal glycation end products within the kidney.
- Obesity targets the kidney by triggering novel pathways of intrarenal inflammation, recruiting professional immunologic cells through so-called metaflammation.
- Obesity-related glomerulopathy has emerged as a distinct pathologic variant of focal segmental glomerulosclerosis.
- No definitive treatments have emerged for obesity-related glomerulopathy, but among the most promising prospects is aggressive weight loss, including bariatric surgery.

EPIDEMIOLOGY OF OBESITY-RELATED KIDNEY DISEASE
Key Points

- Over the past 3 decades, there has been an increase in obesity in the United States, with major costs to the health care system.
- There has been a similar increase in the prevalence of chronic kidney disease (CKD) and end-stage renal disease (ESRD), for both genders, for all adult age ranges, and throughout the developed world.
- There are common factors in both of these phenomena, including hypertension and diabetes.
- Obesity is a powerful risk factor for increased mortality among patients with CKD and ESRD.
- An epidemic of obesity-related kidney disease has been predicted.

[a] Nova Southeastern University, 3200 S. University Drive, Fort Lauderdale, FL 33328, USA; [b] 2150 SE Salerno Rd, Suite 200, Stuart, FL 34997, USA; [c] 200 SE, Hospital Ave. Stuart, FL 34994, USA
* Corresponding author.
E-mail address: snyderdo@nova.edu

Prim Care Clin Office Pract 41 (2014) 875–893
http://dx.doi.org/10.1016/j.pop.2014.08.008   **primarycare.theclinics.com**

The United States is struggling with an epidemic of obesity. According to US Centers for Disease Control and Prevention (CDC) data, in 1988, only about 15% of the American population was obese, defined as body mass index (BMI) greater than 30 kg/m². No state at that time had more than 15% of its adult population classified as obese. This percentage has increased annually, and almost astronomically. As of 2012, more than 25% of the adult population of 42 states was overweight, and in 13 states more than 30% are obese (**Fig. 1**). More than 35% of American adults (78 million) are now obese, as well as 17% of children (12.5 million).[1] The health care costs of obesity are enormous: estimated at $147 billion in 2008. Obese individuals each create an excess $1429 in medical costs annually.[2]

As obesity has increased over the past decade and a half there has been a parallel increase in the prevalence of CKD. This increase has been shown by the United States Renal Data System (USRDS) and National Health and Nutrition Examination Survey (NHANES) data with CKD prevalence rates of 12.3% (1988–1994) up to 14.0% (2005–2010).[3] This increase in CKD prevalence has been observed for every age group, for both genders, for each stage of CKD, and for every ethnic group (although not evenly).[4–6] This increase is an international phenomenon, with similar data having been reported from many developed nations, in which both CKD and obesity prevalence are increasing similarly to the United States.[7]

What is the relationship between obesity and CKD? What factors or comorbidities contribute to this association? According to Framingham data, 78% of hypertension in men and 65% in women is related to excess weight. Furthermore, there is a high degree of correlation between obesity and type 2 diabetes. Diabetes and hypertension are the first and second leading causes of CKD and ESRD. When this information is put together, the increase in ESRD over the last 2 decades mirrors the increase in obesity. This inference is strengthened when leading risk factors are examined together. From the late 1970s throughout the 1990s, smoking, hypertension, and hypercholesterolemia as risk factors for CKD/ESRD were declining, according to USRDS data, whereas prevalence of obesity and ESRD were increasing almost in parallel (**Fig. 2**).[8]

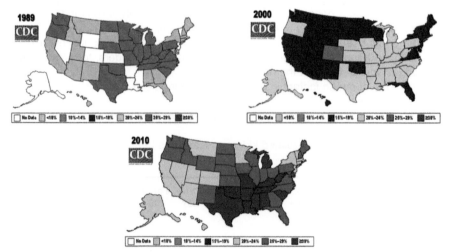

Fig. 1. The increasing incidence of obesity across the United States. (*From* Centers for Disease Control and Prevention. Available at: http://www.cdc.gov/obesity/data/adult.html. Accessed on September 24, 2014.)

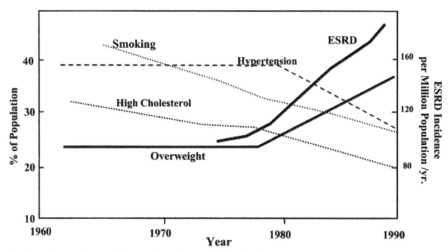

Fig. 2. Estimated prevalence of cardiovascular risk factors as assessed by the NHANES I, II, and III, and incidence of ESRD reported by the United States Renal Data Systems Surveys (USRDS). (*From* Hall JE, Crook ED, Jones DW, et al. Mechanisms of obesity-associated cardiovascular and renal disease. Am J Med Sci 2002;324(3):127–37.)

An even more powerful correlation to consider is the mortality risk, relative to BMI, in individuals with CKD/ESRD. The percentage of individuals with CKD/ESRD and BMI greater than 30 kg/m^2 may seem less than in the population at large, but when the hazard ratio is analyzed, all-cause mortality increases exponentially with incremental increases in BMI (**Fig. 3**).[9] These data suggests that the epidemic increase in obesity has contributed to the smaller epidemic of CKD and subsequent increased incidence of ESRD.

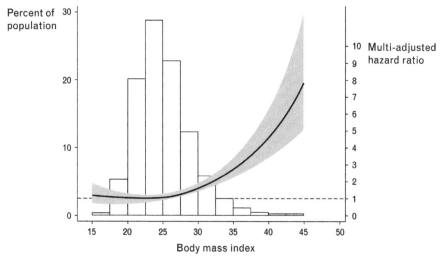

Fig. 3. Hazard ration of death related to BMI versus CKD/ESRD. (*From* Munkhaugen J, Lydersen S, Wideroe TK, et al. Prehypertension, obesity, and risk of kidney disease: 20-year follow-up of the HUNT I study in Norway. Am J Kidney Dis 2009;54(4):638–46.)

GENETICS OF OBESITY-RELATED KIDNEY DISEASE
Key Points

- There are still many unknowns in the understanding of the genetics of obesity and, except for a few conditions, in the understanding of the genetics of CKD.
- It is likely that the most complete understanding of the hereditability of obesity-related kidney disease will be found in the considerations of epigenetic, epigenomic, and environmental factors together.

Extensive research has been conducted on the genetics of obesity, with many strands, but no clear or convincing conclusions yet. Genetic factors are thought to underlie 40% to 90% of prevalent obesity.[10] In 2007, singe-nucleotide polymorphisms (SNPs) were found within a gene known as FTO (fat mass and obesity-associated gene) and these SNPs are associated with human body mass.[11] However, the way these SNPs change or affect weight is still unknown. Factors at play may include neurologic determinants of appetite or whole-body or peripheral pathways of energy expenditure. The specific mechanism of gene activation is not yet known, but there is likely an operative role of both epigenetic and environmental factors. In addition to FTO, leading candidates include the gene coding for the hormone leptin and genes that code for pro-opiomelanocortin (pro-opiomelanocortin correlates the genetic basis for regulation of blood pressure with changes in body weight).[12]

Except for those few conditions with known hereditary pathways (eg, autosomal dominant polycystic kidney disease), there is the same uncertainty regarding genetic, epigenetic, and environmental programming for most types of kidney disease. It is known that kidney disease of several types is associated with polymorphisms of the genes coding angiotensin-converting enzyme (ACE) polymorphisms,[13–15] and ACE polymorphisms seem to be the leading candidates for study of genetic relationships among obesity, kidney disease, and obesity and diabetes or insulin resistance. A survey of international literature shows the influence of the DD allele of the ACE gene, but there is still significant variability in ACE polymorphisms and their relationships to kidney disease.[16–18] Such influence as there might be seems to be generally complex, with other genetic factors at work, as well as epigenetic and environmental factors. It is difficult with the current knowledge to make generalizations across racial or ethnic boundaries.

ACE polymorphisms and genes coding for angiotensin have been similarly implicated in pathogenesis of hypertension, with or without kidney disease, but with inconsistent results. There is similar literature showing the inconsistencies in correlation of ACE polymorphisms with diabetes mellitus and with the metabolic syndrome.[19–25]

More recently the emphasis in research has been to incorporate epigenetic, epigenomic, and environmental considerations in conjunction with interpretation of genetic data.[26–30] It is unlikely that a comprehensive, purely genetic model can be developed to explain the predispositions to obesity, kidney disease, hypertension, and glucose intolerance, as well as racial and ethnic variations of disease. A more comprehensive picture of epigenomic and environmental influences is likely to be needed to accurately display this intricate relationship of disease processes. It could be speculated that environmental and socioeconomic factors may play an essential role in conditioning epigenetic influences on expression of proteinuria, CKD, and obesity-related glomerulopathy (ORG).[31–33]

In short, it seems likely that nurture is at least as powerful as nature, if not more so, when it comes to obesity and its relationship to the kidney.

HYPERTENSION, OBESITY, AND THE KIDNEY
Key Points

- Framingham data show the role of obesity in increasing the prevalence of hypertension.
- Obesity exacerbates hypertension through increased sympathetic nervous system activation, renin-angiotensin-aldosterone activation, and hyperinsulinemia, similar to the mechanisms of CKD.
- Obesity causes salt and water retention and vasoconstriction, exacerbating hypertension.
- Adipocytes are the site of activation of local renin-angiotensin stimulation.

More than 30% of Americans (58 to 65 million) have hypertension.[34] The prevalence of hypertension has been increasing over the past decade as a result of increasing life span and the obesity epidemic. Increased BMI is a strong risk factor for the development of hypertension. As noted earlier, the Framingham Heart Data showed obesity as a pivotal factor leading to incident cases of hypertension at a rate of 26% in men and 28% in women.[35]

The mechanisms by which obesity increases blood pressure are multiple, influenced by both environmental and genetic components. Sodium retention and increased sympathetic activity are essential to the development of hypertension in obese individuals. Sodium retention is a result of increased renal reabsorption of sodium with compromised pressure natriuresis, caused by hyperinsulinemia.[36,37] Sympathetic activity may be increased through several different mechanisms, including activation of the renin-angiotensin-aldosterone system, hyperinsulinemia, obstructive sleep apnea, or alterations in leptin or other adipokines.[36,37]

Lifestyle modifications, including sodium restriction and weight loss, have been shown to help reduce blood pressure in obese patients. The most significant results are seen with weight loss. On average, for each kilogram of weight loss, an individual's blood pressure was reduced by approximately 1 mm Hg.[38]

More than 85% of patients with CKD have hypertension.[39] Patients with obesity and hypertension have an even higher prevalence of CKD compared with individuals with normal BMI. Hypertension not only leads to the development of CKD but hypertension can develop as a result of CKD, leading to further impairments in volume status, in a vicious cycle.

The renal lesion that develops from hypertension is referred to as hypertensive nephrosclerosis. The pathologic findings on histology of patients with hypertensive nephrosclerosis include vascular, glomerular, and tubulointerstitial processes.[40] The obesity-related effects of hypertension may be difficult to separate from hypertensive nephrosclerosis resulting from essential hypertension, until glomerulopathy becomes apparent, as discussed later. Essential hypertension leading to progressive CKD and ESRD has a low incidence rate, unless patients have associated risk factors for progression of renal disease, especially diabetic nephropathy or African American race. Effective blood pressure control typically leads to a slowed progression of renal disease in these patients, with variability in progression attributable to comorbid conditions and, possibly, genetic variability.

GLUCOSE INTOLERANCE, DIABETES, OBESITY
Key Points

- Obesity causes insulin resistance and glucose intolerance through uncertain mechanisms, and contributes to increasing the burden of diabetes.
- Obesity induces advanced glycation end products (AGEs), and AGEs are also ingested at increased rates in the diets of obese individuals.

- AGEs induce soluble receptors (RAGEs), and the AGE-RAGE complex contributes to renal inflammation and glomerular damage.
- Numerous lines of investigation are underway to develop effective therapies to reduce levels of AGEs, inhibit induction of RAGE, or mitigate RAGE-mediated renal injury.

Obesity causes hyperglycemia at least in part through the development of insulin resistance, although the mechanisms behind this are not fully understood. Some studies have observed an imbalance of signal transduction pathways that lead to decreased glucose uptake by the muscle, altered uptake and metabolism of glucose by adipose tissue, and increased glucose output by the liver.[41] Whether or not overt diabetes is present, hyperglycemia associated with obesity has been shown to cause renal damage. A common mechanism of injury is via the development of AGEs. These compounds are produced as a result of nonenzymatic addition of reduced sugar molecules to simple amino acids or proteins in an irreversible Maillard reaction; the browning reaction.[42] This reaction is the same as occurs when dough is baked into bread, as the crust browns; however, in the body, glucose is baked onto cell membranes and other tissues irreversibly. Although AGEs were first identified in diabetes, increased levels of AGEs are present in other conditions as well, such as Alzheimer disease, psoriasis, and obesity. In addition to the endogenous production of AGEs, exogenous AGEs from dietary sources also contribute to their increase in the blood and the induction of specific receptors.[43] Such dietary sources include overconsumption of cooked animal fats and proteins and simple or fructose-based carbohydrates. In animal models, such overfeeding causes glomerular damage in mesangial cells and podocytes, with increased apoptosis and inflammation, mediated by RAGE.[44]

The induction of these RAGEs by AGEs activates an array of signal transduction pathways. In patients with obesity, these receptors can be found in sites of inflammation and as circulating soluble proteins in serum.[45] The resulting AGE-RAGE signaling cascades have been implicated in the damage of many organs including the kidney. The amount of soluble RAGE has been correlated with increased levels of tumor necrosis factor alpha (TNF-α) and other inflammatory molecules, and reactive oxygen species that contribute to renal disease.[46] The AGE-RAGE complex stimulates renal inflammation by stimulation of cytokines, and induces stress and premature senescence by altering signal transduction in the proximal tubule,[47] and AGE also cross-links with collagen to stimulate fibrosis.[48] At least some of the RAGE-induced damage might be related to activation of the renin-angiotensin system glomeruli,[49] which may link this mechanism to obesity-mediated hypertension as well. Although it seems that levels of AGE may portend renal outcome in obesity-related kidney disease, and are implicated in development of generalized atherosclerosis, it is more difficult to use AGE level as a surrogate for renal or cardiovascular outcome.[50]

There are several ways that RAGE-induced damage is being targeted experimentally. In diabetic mice, oat fiber attenuates AGE levels and RAGE-induced cytokine release.[51] A member of the garlic family has been found to reduce AGE formation and cytokine expression.[52] Numerous studies investigate the effects on AGE-RAGE expression of currently used medications. For example, hydralazine has shown reduction of AGEs by protein transglycation (ie, blocking the irreversible step of glycation).[52] peroxisome proliferator-activated receptor γ (PPAR-γ) agonists such as troglitazone and pioglitazone have been found to attenuate RAGE expression.[53] Metformin inhibits AGEs by suppressing generation of reactive oxygen species.[54] Statins may reduce renal tubular injury by inhibiting AGE levels.[55] Novel agents such as human RAGE antibody and pigment epithelium-derived factor show protection against AGE-mediated podocyte injury.[56,57] In addition, diet alone is under investigation, both in humans and animals, with evidence that low-AGE diets might attenuate the development of renal disease.[58] These topics represent only some of the major themes of investigation. At this time, it is not clear which (if any) will emerge as being effective in humans.

INFLAMMATION IN OBESITY-RELATED KIDNEY DISEASE
Key Points

- Obesity is an inflammatory condition.
- Novel pathways of inflammation have been found in the kidney, triggered by obesity.
- The chronic oversupply of nutrients sets up a state, known as metaflammation, in which professional immunologic cells are continuously activated.
- Inflammation is perpetuated by obesity-induced changes in hormonal derangements associated with loss of appetite control, especially leptin.
- Obesity-induced renal inflammation is associated with CKD.

Obesity creates a low-level chronic inflammatory state called metaflammation. It is triggered by an increased metabolic rate as a result of excess consumption of nutrients.[46] Metaflammation has been shown to facilitate the progression of obesity-related diseases, particularly renal disease. The adipocyte plays a key role in the propagation of this condition. The development of metaflammation begins at the intracellular level of the adipocyte. The activity level of several pathways, including c-junctional N-terminal kinase (JNK) and Toll receptor, have been observed to be increased in subjects with obesity and are implicated in the production of inflammation in metabolic tissues.[47,48] These pathways lead to the recruitment of inflammatory cells in metabolic tissues, and activation of these inflammatory cells, which mitigates excess release of inflammatory cytokines (**Fig. 4**).

In normal, nonobese individuals, a nutrient load activates intracellular metabolic pathways and, because digestion and metabolism reach completion, no inflammation occurs. However, in overnutrition, metabolic pathways are saturated, and the excessive nutrient load entering the system stimulates pathogen-sensing pathways of the immune system, possibly because nutrients are biological molecules. These inflammatory pathways may block the metabolism of excess nutrients, leading to their storage in adipocytes. As the condition of nutrient excess persists and continues to an extreme, the immune response graduates from the acute pathogen-sensing pathways to the recruitment of professional immune cells. This further inhibits normal nutrient metabolism, encourages storage as adipose tissue, and leads to stimulation and maintenance of chronic inflammation (**Fig. 5**).[46]

Serum levels of inflammatory markers, including TNF-α, interleukin (IL)-6, macrophage inhibitory factor, and other cytokines increase as a result of a chronic oversupply of nutrients. These proinflammatory compounds are either directly produced by adipose cells or by nonfat cells (eg, recruited macrophages) that infiltrate adipose tissue.[50] Called adipocytokines, they have been implicated in various diseases associated with obesity, including renal disease.

TNF-α is a proinflammatory cytokine that is secreted by helper T lymphocytes, B lymphocytes, natural killer cells, macrophages, and nonlymphoid cells. It is an essential component of an array of different inflammatory pathways and plays a key role in the pathology of various inflammatory diseases. In obesity, TNF-α is produced principally by macrophages that have infiltrated adipose tissue. One proposed mechanism of TNF-α–mediated renal disease is that it causes insulin resistance by disrupting signal transduction at the level of the insulin receptor substrate (IRS). TNF-α activates

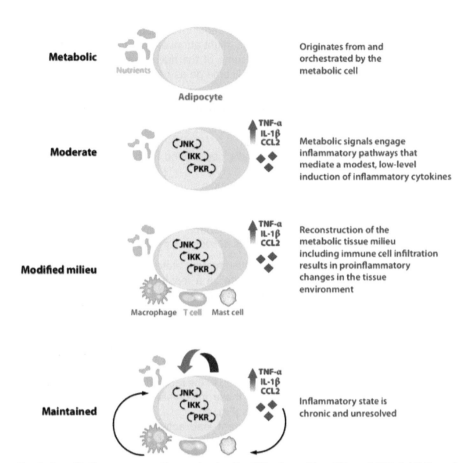

Fig. 4. Renal inflammatory pathways in obesity. CCL, chemokine C ligand; IKK, inhibitor of kappa kinase; IL, interleukin; PKR, protein kinase R. (*From* Gregor MF, Hotamisligil GS. Inflammatory mechanisms in obesity. Annu Rev Immunol 2011;29:415–45; with permission.)

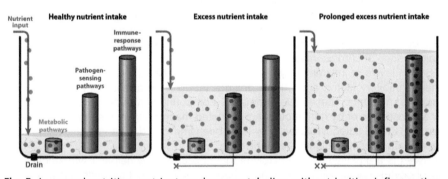

Fig. 5. In normal nutrition, nutrients undergo metabolism without inciting inflammation. Overload of nutrients signal immune pathogen-sensing pathways, and block normal metabolic pathways. If allowed to persist and increase, overnutrition recruits professional immune cells, stimulating ongoing inflammation, blocking normal metabolism, and leading to increased adipose storage and metaflammation. (*From* Gregor MF, Hotamisligil GS. Inflammatory mechanisms in obesity. Annu Rev Immunol 2011;29:415–45; with permission.)

p53 mitogen-activated protein kinase and inhibitor kappa B, leading to phosphorylation of the IRS, which in turn leads to insulin resistance.[51] Multiple mechanisms of renal disease as a result of increased TNF-α expression have been described. TNF-α has been shown to increase renal cellular protein formation (ie, Klotho protein); decrease fibrinolysis, resulting in renal fibrosis; and recruit monocytes. All these pathways lead directly to renal damage.[52–54]

IL-6 is another proinflammatory cytokine that is increased in patients with obesity. In those without obesity, IL-6 is predominantly secreted by T cells and macrophages. In obese individuals this cytokine is also produced directly by adipose tissue when it has been infiltrated by macrophages. IL-6 levels have been shown to correlate directly with BMI.[55] In extremely obese patients with normal kidney function, IL-6 levels correlated with the number of glomerular lesions found on kidney biopsy.[56] Renal biopsies taken from patients with obesity-related renal disease were found to have increased expression of IL-6 signal transduction, further implicating IL-6 in the pathophysiology of obesity-related renal disease.[57]

Systemic inflammation is also influenced by numerous hormones secreted by adipose tissue. Leptin is a hormone produced predominantly by fat cells that serves as a regulator of metabolism and hunger: the satiety hormone. Leptin binds to its receptors in the hypothalamus to produce satiety and increase body temperature.[58] Obesity leads to leptin resistance and hyperleptinemia, both of which lead to damage of multiple organ systems, including the kidney. One of the many mechanisms by which leptin directly or indirectly mediates renal disease is its effect on inflammation. Leptin regulates the secretion of many cytokines, in vitro, including interferon gamma, IL-2, and IL-4. In vivo studies have also associated leptin with increased IL-6 production.[59]

Adiponectin is another complex compound involved in the regulation of inflammation. This hormone is exclusively secreted by adipose tissue, and suppresses the inflammatory response. There is an inverse correlation between adiponectin and each of the following: high sensitivity- C-reactive protein, IL-6, and TNF-α.[60] Adiponectin is found in lower concentrations in patients with obesity, perpetuating and exacerbating chronic low levels of inflammatory activity.

PATHOLOGY OF OBESITY-RELATED KIDNEY DISEASE
Key Points

- The glomerulus is the principal target of obesity-induced inflammation in the kidney.
- The glomerulopathy of ORG is a variant of focal segmental glomerulosclerosis and presents with proteinuria and lipid abnormalities, as with classic nephrotic syndrome.
- Despite the role of insulin resistance and abnormal glycation in pathogenesis of ORG, this is pathologically distinct from diabetic nephropathy.

The principal renal target of obesity is the glomerulus. One of the first comprehensive descriptions of ORG was published in 2001. This retrospective report reviewed renal biopsies from 1986 to 2000. In addition to describing the pathologic features of ORG, the increasing prevalence of the findings was also shown. During this 15-year period, 103 cases of ORG were found in a sample of 6818 biopsies. For the first 5 years of that period, only 2 cases were identified; 77 cases were identified in the last 5 years. The investigators anticipate an incidence of ORG increasing to epidemic proportions, based on the increasing prevalence of obesity.[61]

These biopsies had enough correlation with the classic description of idiopathic focal segmental glomerulosclerosis (FSGS) to warrant categorization as a subset of that entity. Typical histologic findings include segmental increase in basement membrane–like material in the mesangium, variable degrees of glomerular sclerosis, segmental adhesion of the glomerular tuft to the Bowman capsule, variable degrees of tubular atrophy and interstitial fibrosis, and variable degrees of proximal tubular damage. A recent finding, potentially specific to ORG, is proximal tubule epithelial hypertrophy, conceivably related to glomerular hyperfiltration.[62] There are no specific immunofluorescent findings in ORG. On electron microscopy, there are no electron-dense deposits, and podocyte foot processes are effaced. Underlying pathophysiology of these findings has been attributed to glomerular hyperfiltration, insulin resistance, salt sensitivity, hyperactivity of the renin-angiotensin axis, excessive aldosterone, excessive stimulation by cortisol, adiponectin deficiency,[63] deposition of abnormal glycation end products,[64] and other factors. Adiponectin in particular has insulin-sensitizing, antiatherogenic, and antiinflammatory properties. Low concentrations of adiponectin are associated with greater glomerular oxidant stress, albuminuria, as well as cardiovascular risk.[65,66] Mesangial inflammation has been associated with abnormalities in lymphocyte function[67,68] and exhaustion of IL-6.[69] Mild diabetoid changes have been noted that link ORG to diabetic nephropathy, probably through the mechanism of AGE-RAGE interaction, but distinguished from frank diabetic nephropathy by their lesser frequency and intensity.[70] Typical biopsies are shown in **Fig. 6**.

Lesions of podocytes are more pronounced in ORG and may have increased functional significance compared with idiopathic FSGS and diabetic nephropathy. Podocytes are decreased in number and density, with markedly increased foot process width and vacuolization of cytoplasm. These podocyte changes correlate with declining glomerular filtration rate, increasing proteinuria, and insulin resistance. Mesangial changes are not associated with insulin resistance or the degree of proteinuria.[71,72]

Compared with patients with idiopathic FSGS in the series discussed earlier, patients with ORG are younger and heavier. Mean BMI in the study discussed earlier was 41.7 kg/m^2 (range, 30.9–62.7 kg/m^2). There was a moderate male predominance in both series (1.6–2:1). In the American series, there was a great predominance of white patients compared with idiopathic FSGS, for which African American ethnicity is a significant risk factor. Although one-eighth of the patients in this series had diabetes, none had characteristic findings of diabetic nephropathy on biopsy. Proteinuria tends to be less massive in ORG than idiopathic FSGS, with many patients having subnephrotic proteinuria, and far fewer patients having full-blown nephrotic syndrome.

Apart from obesity, a study of numerous metabolic markers found that insulin resistance was predictive of ORG. However, in a binary logistic regression analysis, none of the following were predictive, despite being highly prevalent among patients with obesity and metabolic syndrome: amylin, triglyceride, total cholesterol, high-density lipoprotein (HDL) cholesterol, low-density lipoprotein cholesterol, triglyceride/HDL ratio, fasting glucose, or fasting insulin.[73]

Table 1 summarizes the pathologic distinctions between ORG, idiopathic FSGS, and diabetic nephropathy. In general, weight loss seems to ameliorate proteinuria and slow progression toward ESRD in ORG.[74] There have been some case reports and series attesting that weight loss, either by diet alone[75] or by bariatric surgery, is also associated with pathologic improvement.[76]

TREATMENT
Key Points

- Optimal therapy for obesity-related kidney disease has not yet been defined.
- Despite the role of inflammation in pathogenesis, antiinflammatory therapy has not yet shown benefit.

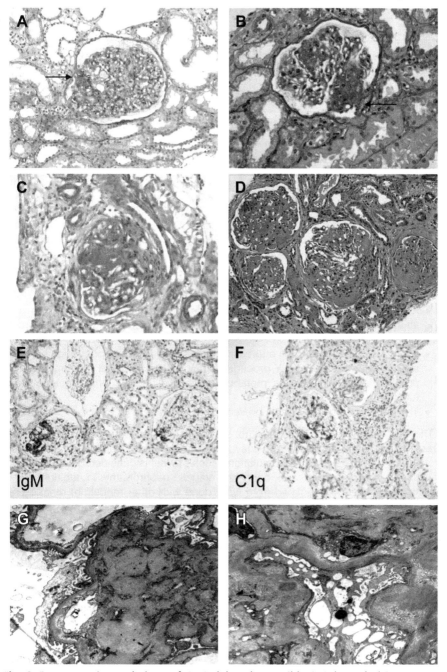

Fig. 6. Representative pathology of ORG. (*A*) Early or mild FSGS (*arrow*). (*B*) FSGS with capillaries adherent to the Bowman capsule (*arrow*). (*C*) FSGS progresses, with obliteration of capillary lumens and development of global sclerosis. (*D*) FSGS with glomerulomegaly. (*E*) Atypical immunohistochemistry staining for immunoglobulin M (IgM). (*F*) Atypical immuno-histochemistry staining for C1q. (*G*) Electron microscopy with increased mesangial matrix, variable glomerular basement membrane thickening, and degenerative changes of podo-cytes. (*H*) Podocyte degenerative processes are variable. (*From* Amman K, Benz K. Structural renal changes in obesity and diabetes. Semin Nephrol 2013;33(1):23–33.)

Table 1
Qualitative general comparison of pathologic features of ORG, idiopathic FSGS, and diabetic nephropathy (DMN)

	ORG	FSGS	DMN
Nephrotic proteinuria	±	+	+
Nephrotic syndrome	±	+	+
Tubulointerstitial changes	+	±	±
Podocyte depletion, expansion	+	+	+
Nodular sclerosis	±	−	+
Glomerulomegaly	+	−	±
Arteriolosclerosis	+	−	±
Immunofluorescent findings	−	−	−
Electron-dense deposits	−	−	−

±, inconsistently present, or not diagnostic.

- Therapies that reduce cross-linking of abnormal glycation end products have been proposed, but have not yet shown benefit.
- As with many other renal diseases, blockade of the renin-angiotensin system and statins may have benefit in reducing proteinuria and mitigating glomerular damage.
- Weight loss, either through aggressive dietary management or through bariatric surgery with the Roux-en-Y procedure, may benefit the renal inflammation and proteinuria, as well as the metabolic milieu of obesity, and preserve renal function.
- The best strategy is probably prevention of obesity.

The best treatment of ORG has not yet been defined. Investigation has been directed toward the pathways of kidney injury, such as the inflammation of obesity, proteinuria, and AGE-RAGE accumulation. Much of what is considered here is based on animal research and on work done with diabetic nephropathy. In addition, some investigations have extrapolated from work done with other models of renal injury, based on common aspects of inflammation, oxidation, and abnormal glycation. These processes are linked, because inflammation causes the generation of oxidative processes that in turn facilitate the generation, cross-linking, and deposition of AGEs.[77]

Pathways of renal inflammation have been targeted in several ways. A recent Cochrane Review examined the role of antioxidants in CKD. In studies on vitamin C, vitamin E, coenzyme Q-10, superoxide dismutase, and acetylcysteine there was no clear benefit in either cardiovascular or renal outcomes. The possibility that antioxidant therapy might slow progression of CKD to ESRD has not yet been resolved, but evidence for the agents listed earlier is not encouraging.[78]

There have been proposed antiinflammatory mechanisms of commonly used medications, such as pioglitazone and pentoxifylline, which may have a role in controlling ORG in the future. In addition to its effect of reducing hyperglycemia in diabetes, pioglitazone seems to have the additional benefits of reducing renal oxidation and downregulating PPAR-γ.[79] Pentoxifylline seems to have favorable effects on inflammation in diabetic nephropathy, reducing albuminuria and preserving creatinine clearance.[80]

Bardoxolone methyl is an agent that was under study for its antiinflammatory effects on the novel Nrf2 pathway in diabetic kidney disease; initial studies were promising, but phase 3 trials were stopped because of a higher-than-expected rate of cardiovascular events.[81] The plant-derived digestive enzyme trigonelline seems to work on the same pathway, and initial reports of its efficacy are encouraging.[82,83]

Statins have been examined for effects on glomerular function in obesity beyond lowering cholesterol. Statins have a positive effect on glomerular inflammation, reducing lipid oxidation, inhibiting thrombogenesis, and preserving podocyte function in obesity, diabetes, and hypertension.[84–86]

Chloroquine has emerged as a potential therapy because of its role in increasing nitric oxide and enhancing glomerular perfusion.[87]

Prevention against AGE-associated damage has been targeted in several ways. Aminoguanidine has been under investigation for several models of kidney disease because of its actions as a nitric oxide synthase inhibitor as well as inhibiting or breaking AGE cross-links; however, it is not under active development for human use at this time.[88,89] Pyridoxamine has been shown to reduce the concentrations of several mediators of inflammation, decrease microalbuminuria, and improve the pathologic appearance of animal kidneys.[90,91] One of the more promising compounds under investigation is alagebrium, which reduces glomerular inflammation and fibrosis, reduces proteinuria, and seems to preserve renal function by breaking AGE cross-links.[92,93]

The most obvious and, arguably, the most important therapeutic question concerns the effect of weight loss on ORG. Although this has not been systematically investigated, there have been several reports suggesting the benefit of bariatric surgery or weight loss by diet.

Weight loss drugs alone do not seem to be the answer. Rimonabant showed some promise of benefit, but has been withdrawn from study.[94] Orlistat is associated with progressive CKD.[95] Sibutramine is unlikely to cause enough weight loss to have any impact.[75] Weight loss by diet has been shown to improve ORG in case reports[73] and small series.[96]

Several reports describe the benefit of bariatric surgery on proteinuria, renal function, and even on glomerular disorders, as well as on the metabolic syndrome. These improvements are associated with Roux-en-Y gastric bypass but not with restrictive procedures such as gastric banding.[97–99]

Therapeutics for ORG are evolving, as summarized in **Table 2**. It is reasonable to apply certain basic principles: blood pressure control, especially with ACE inhibitor or angiotensin receptor blockade; glycemic control, with consideration to include pioglitazone; statins; and weight reduction with diet and/or bariatric surgery. Overall management strategies should target comorbid conditions. The potential benefits of antioxidant or antiinflammatory therapy must be considered to be speculative at this time.

Table 2	
Treatment options for obesity-related kidney disease	
Recommended	**Experimental**
ACE/ARB	Antioxidants
Statin	Vitamin therapy
Glycemic control, consider TZD	Antiinflammatory
Weight loss	NO synthase inhibitor
Bariatric surgery, especially Roux-en-Y	Inhibitors of glycation end-product cross-linking

Abbreviations: ARB, angiotensin receptor blocker; TZD, thiazolidinedione.

SUMMARY

As the epidemic of obesity continues to increase, ORG will become an even greater problem. As clinicians gain greater insight into the pathophysiology of obesity and its related issues, including ORG, hypertension, and insulin resistance, it is hoped that new and better tools will be developed to treat it. Weight loss must be at the cornerstone of any therapeutic edifice. Prevention of obesity and ORG is even more important and effective than any treatment. Patients should be counseled that they can out-eat the benefits of any medication and no medication is more powerful than prevention of obesity through proper principles of diet and physical activity.

REFERENCES

1. Freedman D. Obesity—United States, 1988–2008. MMWR Surveill Summ 2011; 60(1):73–7.
2. Centers for Disease Control and Prevention. Overweight and obesity: adult obesity facts. Available at: http://www.cdc.gov/obesity/data/adult.html. Accessed on September 24, 2014.
3. United States Renal Data System. 2013 Atlas of CKD and ESRD [Chapter 1]. 2013. p. 44–50. Available at: http://www.usrds.org/adr.aspx. Accessed on September 24, 2014.
4. Coresh J, Selvin E, Stevens WA, et al. Prevalence of chronic kidney disease in the United States. JAMA 2007;298(17):2038–47.
5. Glassock RJ, Winearls C. An epidemic of chronic kidney disease: fact or fiction? Nephrol Dial Transplant 2008;23(4):1117–21.
6. USRDS 2004 report. Available at: http://www.usrds.org/atlas04/aspx. Accessed on September 24, 2014.
7. Zoccali C, Kramer A, Jager KJ. Epidemiology of CKD in Europe: an uncertain scenario. Nephrol Dial Transplant 2010;25(6):1731–3.
8. Hall JE, Crook ED, Jones DW, et al. Mechanisms of obesity-associated cardiovascular and renal disease. Am J Med Sci 2002;324(3):127–37.
9. Munkhaugen J, Lydersen S, Wideroe TK, et al. Pre-hypertension, obesity and risk of kidney disease: 20-year follow-up of the HUNT-1 study in Norway. Am J Kidney Dis 2009;54(4):638–46.
10. Maes HH, Neale MC, Eaves LJ. Genetic and environmental factors in relative body weight and human adiposity. Behav Genet 2008;27:325–51.
11. Fawcett KA, Barroso I. The genetics of obesity: FTO leads the way. Trends Genet 2010;26:266–74.
12. Ramachandrappa S, Farooqi IS. Genetic approaches to understanding human obesity. J Clin Invest 2011;121(6):2080–6.
13. Elshamaa MF, Sabty SM, Bazaara HM, et al. Genetic polymorphism of ACE and the angiotensin II type 1 receptor genes in children with chronic kidney disease. J Inflamm 2011;8(1):20.
14. Campbell CY, Fang BF, Guo X, et al. Associations between genetic variants in the ACE, AGT, AGTR1 and AGTR2 genes and renal function in the Multiethnic Study of Atherosclerosis. Am J Nephrol 2010;32(2):156–62.
15. Rudnicki M, Mayer G. Significance of genetic polymorphisms of the renin-angiotensin-aldosterone system in cardiovascular and renal disease. Pharmacogenomics 2009;10(3):463–76.
16. Bell CG, Meyre D, Petretto E, et al. No contribution of angiotensin-converting enzyme gene variants to severe obesity: a model for comprehensive

case/control and quantitative cladistics analysis of ACE in human diseases. Eur J Hum Genet 2007;15(3):320–7.

17. Su SL, Lu KC, Lin YF, et al. Gene polymorphisms of angiotensin-converting enzyme and angiotensin II type 1 receptor among chronic kidney disease patients in a Chinese population. J Renin Angiotensin Aldosterone Syst 2012; 13(1):148–54.

18. Gui-Yan QW, Yan-hua W, Qun X, et al. Associations between RAS gene polymorphisms, environmental factors and hypertension in Mongolian people. Eur J Epidemiol 2006;21(4):287–92.

19. Mehri S, Jahjoub S, Hammami S, et al. Renin-angiotensin system polymorphisms in relation to hypertension status and obesity in a Tunisian population. Mol Biol Rep 2012;39(4):4059–65.

20. Siklar Z, Berberoglu M, Savas Erdeve S, et al. Contribution of clinical, metabolic and genetic factors on hypertension in obese children and adolescents. J Pediatr Endocrinol Metab 2011;24(1–2):21–4.

21. Mittal G, Gupta V, Haque SF, et al. Effect of angiotensin converting enzyme gene I/D polymorphism in patients with metabolic syndrome in North Indian population. Chin Med J 2011;124(1):45–8.

22. Fiatal S, Szigethy E, Szeles G, et al. Insertion/deletion polymorphism of angiotensin-1 converting enzyme is associated with metabolic syndrome in Hungarian adults. J Renin Angiotensin Aldosterone Syst 2011;12(4):531–8.

23. Mondry A, Loh M, Liu P, et al. Polymorphisms of the insertion/deletion ACE and M235T AGT genes and hypertension: surprising new findings and met-analysis of date. BMC Nephrol 2005;6:1.

24. Procopciuc LM, Sitar-Taut A, Pop D, et al. Renin angiotensin system polymorphisms in patients with metabolic syndrome. Eur J Intern Med 2010;21(5): 414–8.

25. Thomas GN, Tomlinson B, Chan JC, et al. Renin-angiotensin system gene polymorphisms, blood pressure, dyslipidemia, and diabetes in Hong Kong Chinese: a significant association of the ACE insertion/deletions polymorphism with type 2 diabetes. Diabetes Care 2001;24(2):356–61.

26. Toubal A, Treuter E, Clement K, et al. Genomic and epigenetic regulation of adipose tissue inflammation in obesity. Trends Endocrinol Metab 2013;24(12): 625–34.

27. Amarasekera M, Prescott SL, Palmer DJ. Nutrition in early life, immune-programming and allergies: the role of epigenetics. Asian Pac J Allergy Immunol 2013;31(3):175–82.

28. Tiwari S, Ndisang JF. The role of obesity in cardiomyopathy and nephropathy. Curr Pharm Des 2014;20(9):1409–17.

29. Houde AA, Hivert MF, Bouchard L. Fetal epigenetic programming of adipokines. Adipocyte 2013;2(1):41–6.

30. Dwivedi RS, Herman JG, McCaffrey TA, et al. Beyond genetics: epigenetic code in chronic kidney disease. Kidney Int 2011;79(1):23–32.

31. Martins D, Tareen N, Zadshir A, et al. Association of poverty with the prevalence of albuminuria: data from the third National Health and Nutrition Examination Survey (NHANES III). Am J Kidney Dis 2006;47(6):965–71.

32. Ali MK, Bullard KM, Beckles GL, et al. Household income and cardiovascular disease risks in U.S. children and young adults. Diabetes Care 2011;34(9): 1998–2004.

33. Lakkis J, Wier M. Pharmacological strategies for kidney function preservation: are there differences by ethnicity? Adv Ren Replace Ther 2004;11(1):24–40.

34. Egan BM, Zhao Y, Axon RN. US trends in prevalence, awareness, treatment, and control of hypertension, 1988–2008. JAMA 2010;303(20):2043.

35. Wilson PW, D'Agostino RP, Sullivan L, et al. Overweight and obesity as determinants of cardiovascular risk: the Framingham experience. Arch Intern Med 2002;162:1867–72.

36. Kotchen TA. Obesity-related hypertension: epidemiology, pathophysiology, and clinical management. Am J Hypertens 2010;23(11):1170–8.

37. Montani JP, Antic V, Yang Z, et al. Pathways from obesity to hypertension: from the perspective of a vicious triangle. Int J Obes Relat Metab Disord 2002; 26(Suppl 2):s28–38.

38. Aucott L, Rothnie H, McIntyre L, et al. Long-term weight loss from lifestyle intervention benefits blood pressure? A systematic review. Hypertension 2009;54: 756–62.

39. Whaley-Connell AT, Sowers JR, Stevens LA, et al. CKD in the United States: Kidney Early Evaluation Program (KEEP) and National Health and Nutrition Examination Survey (NHANES) 1999-2004. Am J Kidney Dis 2008; 51(4 Suppl 2):S13.

40. Freedman BI, Iskandar SS, Appel RG. The link between hypertension and nephrosclerosis. Am J Kidney Dis 1995;25(2):207.

41. Martyn J, Kaneki M, Yasuhara S. Obesity-induced insulin resistance and hyperglycemia: etiological factors and molecular mechanisms. Anesthesiology 2008; 109(1):137–48.

42. Tomino Y, Hagiwara S, Gohda T. AGE-RAGE interaction and oxidative stress in obesity-related renal dysfunction. Kidney Int 2011;80(2):133–5.

43. Sparvero LJ, Asafu-Adjei D, Kang R. RAGE (receptor for advanced glycation endproducts), RAGE ligands, and their role in cancer and inflammation. J Transl Med 2009;7:17.

44. Tan AL, Forbes JM, Cooper ME. AGE RAGE, and ROS in diabetic nephropathy. Semin Nephrol 2007;27(2):130–43.

45. Gregor M, Hotamisligil G. Inflammatory mechanisms in obesity. Annu Rev Immunol 2011;29:415–45.

46. Solinas G, Karin M. JNK1 and IKKbeta: molecular links between obesity and metabolic dysfunction. FASEB J 2010;24(8):2596–611.

47. Shi H, Kokoeva MV, Inouye K, et al. TLR4 links innate immunity and fatty acid-induced insulin resistance. J Clin Invest 2006;116(11):739–45.

48. Marjolein V, Bouter L, McQuillan G, et al. Elevated C-reactive protein levels in overweight and obese adults. JAMA 1999;282(22):2131–5.

49. Fain JN, Bahouth SW, Madan AK. TNFalpha release by the nonfat cells of human adipose tissue. Int J Obes Relat Metab Disord 2004;28(4):616–22.

50. Nieto-Vasquez I, Fernandez-velido S, Kramer DK, et al. Insulin resistance associated to obesity: the link TNF alpha. Arch Physiol Biochem 2008;114(3):183–94.

51. Moreno JA, Izquierdo MC, Sanchez-Nino MD, et al. The inflammatory cytokines TWEAK and TNFα reduce renal klotho expression through NFκB. J Am Soc Nephrol 2011;22(7):1315–25.

52. Rerolle JP, Hertig A, Nguyen G, et al. Plasminogen activator inhibitor type 1 is a potential target in renal fibrogenesis. Kidney Int 2000;58(5):1841–50.

53. Matoba K, Kawanami D, Ishizawa S, et al. Rho-kinase mediates TNF-α-induced MCP-1 expression via p38 MAPK signaling pathway in mesangial cells. Biochem Biophys Res Commun 2010;402(4):725–30.

54. Roytblat L, Rachinsky M, Fisher A, et al. Raised interleukin-6 levels in obese patients. Obes Res 2000;8(9):673–5.

55. Serra A, Romero R, Lopez D, et al. Renal injury in the extremely obese patients with normal renal function. Kidney Int 2008;73(8):947–55.
56. Wu Y, Liu Z, Xiang Z, et al. Obesity-related glomerulopathy: insights from gene expression profiles of the glomeruli derived from renal biopsy samples. Endocrinology 2006;147(1):44–50.
57. Lord GM, Matarese G, Howard JK, et al. Leptin modulates the T-cell immune response and reverses starvation-induced immunosuppression. Nature 1998; 394(6696):897–901.
58. Agnello D, Meazza C, Rowan CG, et al. Leptin causes body weight loss in the absence of in vivo activities typical of cytokines of the IL-6 family. Am J Physiol 1998;275(3 pt 2):R913–9.
59. Engeli S, Feldpausch M, Gorzelniak K, et al. Association between adiponectin and mediators of inflammation in obese women. Diabetes 2003;52(4):942–7.
60. Kambham N, Markowitz GS, Valeri AM, et al. Obesity-related glomerulopathy: an emerging epidemic. Kidney Int 2001;59:1498–509.
61. Tobar A, Ori Y, Benchetrit S, et al. Proximal tubular hypertrophy and enlarged glomerular and proximal tubular urinary space in obese subjects with proteinuria. PLoS One 2013;8(9):e75547.
62. Amann K, Benz K. Structural renal changes in obesity and diabetes. Semin Nephrol 2013;33(1):23–33.
63. D'Agati V, Schmidt AM. RAGE and the pathogenesis of chronic kidney disease. Nat Rev Nephrol 2010;6(6):352–60.
64. Shen YY, Peake PW, Charlesworth JA. Adiponectin: its role in kidney disease. Nephrology (Carlton) 2008;13:528–34.
65. Sharma K. The link between obesity and albuminuria: adiponectin and podocyte dysfunction. Kidney Int 2009;76(2):145–8.
66. Chatzigeorgiou A, Karalis KP, Bornsteint SR, et al. Lymphocytes in obesity-related adipose tissue inflammation. Diabetologia 2012;55(10):2583–92.
67. Gotoh K, Inoue M, Masaki T, et al. Obesity-related chronic kidney disease is associated with spleen-derived IL-10. Nephrol Dial Transplant 2013;28(5): 1120–30.
68. Harcourt BE, Forbes JM, Matthews VB. Obesity-induced renal impairment is exacerbated in interleukin-6 knockout mice. Nephrology (Carlton) 2012;17(3): 257–62.
69. Darouich S, Goucha R, Jaafoura MH, et al. Clinicopathological characteristics of obesity-associated focal segmental glomerulosclerosis. Ultrastruct Pathol 2011; 35(4):176–82.
70. Chen HM, Liu ZH, Zeng CH, et al. Podocyte lesions in patients with obesity-related glomerulopathy. Am J Kidney Dis 2006;48(5):772–9.
71. Tsuboi N, Utsunomiya Y, Kanzaki G, et al. Low glomerular density with glomerulomegaly in obesity-related glomerulopathy. Clin J Am Soc Nephrol 2012;7(5): 735–41.
72. Chen HM, Li SJ, Chen HP, et al. Obesity-related glomerulopathy in China: a case series of 90 patients. Am J Kidney Dis 2008;52(1):58–65.
73. Shen WW, Chen HM, Chen H, et al. Obesity-related glomerulopathy: body mass index and proteinuria. Clin J Am Soc Nephrol 2010;5(8):1401–9.
74. Fowler SM, Kon V, Ma L, et al. Obesity-related focal and segmental glomerulosclerosis: normalization of proteinuria in an adolescent after bariatric surgery. Pediatr Nephrol 2009;24(4):851–5.
75. Tran HA. Reversible obesity-related glomerulopathy following weight reduction. Med J Aust 2006;184(7):367.

76. Engelen L, Stehouwer DC, Schalkwijk CG. Current therapeutic interventions in the glycation pathway: evidence from clinical studies. Diabetes Obes Metab 2013;15(8):677–89.
77. Jun M, Venkataraman V, Razavian M, et al. Antioxidants for chronic kidney disease. Cochrane Database Syst Rev 2012;(10):CD008176.
78. Hirasawa Y, Matsui Y, Yamane K, et al. Pioglitazone improves obesity type diabetic nephropathy: relation to the mitigation of renal oxidative reaction. Exp Anim 2008;57(5):423–32.
79. Shan D, Wu HM, Yuan QY, et al. Pentoxifylline for diabetic kidney disease. Cochrane Database Syst Rev 2012;(2):CD006800.
80. De Zeeuw D, Akizawa T, Audhya P, et al. Bardoxolone methyl in type 2 diabetes and stage 4 chronic kidney disease. N Engl J Med 2013;369:2493–503.
81. Hamden K, Mnafgui K, Amri Z, et al. Inhibition of key digestive enzymes related to diabetes and hyperlipidemia and protection of liver-kidney function by trigonelline in diabetic rats. Sci Pharm 2013;81(1):233–46.
82. Ghule AE, Jadhav SS, Bodhankar SL. Trigonelline ameliorates diabetic hypertensive nephropathy by suppression of oxidative stress in kidney and reduction in renal cell apoptosis and fibrosis in streptozotocin induced neonatal diabetic rats. Int Immunopharmacol 2012;14(4):740–8.
83. Knight SF, Yuan J, Roy S, et al. Simvastatin and tempol protect against endothelial dysfunction and renal injury in a model of obesity and hypertension. Am J Physiol Renal Physiol 2010;298(1):F86–94.
84. Whaley-Connell A, DeMarco VG, Lastra G, et al. Insulin resistance, oxidative stress, and podocyte injury: role of rosuvastatin in modulation of filtration barrier injury. Am J Nephrol 2008;28(1):67–75.
85. Wei J, Ma C, Wang X. Simvastatin inhibits tissue factor and plasminogen activator inhibitor-1 expression of glomerular mesangial cells in hypercholesterolemic rabbits. Biomed Res 2006;27(4):149–55.
86. Osman MM, Khalil A, Ahmed MH. Chloroquine-induced nitric oxide: new treatment for an emerging epidemic of obesity-related glomerulopathy. Diabetes Technol Ther 2006;8(6):691–2.
87. El Shazly AH, Mahmoud AM, Darwish NS. Potential prophylactic role of aminoguanidine in diabetic retinopathy and nephropathy in experimental animals. Acta Pharm 2009;59(1):67–73.
88. Abdel-Rahman E, Bolton WK. Pimagedine: a novel therapy for diabetic nephropathy. Expert Opin Investig Drugs 2002;11(4):565–74.
89. Elseweldy MM, Elswefy SE, Younis NN, et al. Pyridoxamine, an inhibitor of protein glycation, in relation to microalbuminuria and proinflammatory cytokines in experimental diabetic nephropathy. Exp Biol Med 2013;238(8):881–8.
90. Nakamura S, Li H, Adijiang A. Pyridoxal phosphate prevents progression of diabetic nephropathy. Nephrol Dial Transplant 2007;22(8):2165–74.
91. Waston AM, Gray SP, Jiaze L, et al. Alagebrium reduces glomerular fibrogenesis and inflammation beyond preventing RAGE activation in diabetic apolipoprotein E knockout mice. Diabetes 2012;61(8):2105–13.
92. Park J, Kwon MK, Huh JY, et al. Renoprotective antioxidant effect of alagebrium in experimental diabetes. Nephrol Dial Transplant 2011;26(11):3473–84.
93. Ahmed MH. Rimonabant as a potential new treatment for an emerging epidemic of obesity-related glomerulopathy? Expert Opin Emerg Drugs 2006;11(4):563–5.
94. Coutinho AK, Glancey GR. Orlistat, an under-recognised cause of progressive renal impairment. Nephrol Dial Transplant 2013;28(Suppl 4):172–4, iv.

95. Veerman JL, Barendregt JJ, Forster M, et al. Cost-effectiveness of pharmaco-therapy to reduce obesity. PLoS One 2011;6(10):e26051.
96. Serpa Neto A, Bianco Rossi FM, Dal Moro Amarante R, et al. Effect of weight loss after Roux-en-Y gastric bypass on renal function and blood pressure in morbidly obese patients. J Nephrol 2009;22(5):637–46.
97. Huan Y, Tomaszewski JE, Cohen DL. Resolution of nephrotic syndrome after successful bariatric surgery in patient with biopsy proven FSGS. Clin Nephrol 2009;71(1):69–73.
98. Alexander JW, Goodman HR, Hawver LR, et al. Improvement and stabilization of chronic kidney disease after gastric bypass. Surg Obes Relat Dis 2009;5(2):237–41.
99. Fenske W, Athanasiou T, Harling L, et al. Obesity-related cardiorenal disease: the benefits of bariatric surgery. Nat Rev Nephrol 2013;9:539–51.

Medical Management of the Kidney Transplant Recipient

A Practical Approach for the Primary Care Provider

Fernando Pedraza, MD, David Roth, MD*

KEYWORDS

- Kidney transplant recipient • Hypertension • Diabetes • Obesity • Dyslipidemia

KEY POINTS

- Kidney transplant recipients (KTR) commonly present with a multitude of metabolic derangements that have a major impact on long-term outcomes.
- The successful management of the KTR requires a collaborative effort between the primary care physician and the transplant center.
- Hypertension is present in more than 80% of these patients and often requires multiple medications to achieve the established, aggressive systolic and diastolic targets.
- Diabetes mellitus can be present before transplant or occur as a de novo medical issue in the posttransplant period. Corticosteroids and other immunosuppressives are contributory.
- Dyslipidemia and obesity are challenging problems commonly encountered in the medical management of the KTR and require effective treatment strategies on a long-term basis.

INTRODUCTION

Evolving trends in health care have placed the primary care physician (PCP) at the forefront of long-term patient management. Not infrequently, PCPs are required to manage and make clinical decisions with patients with complex medical conditions that are not in disciplines for which they have received formal training. An example of this is the kidney transplant recipient (KTR), a patient that commonly has multiple comorbidities, including hypertension (HTN), diabetes mellitus, dyslipidemia, and obesity. This is on a background of end-stage renal disease further complicated by the complexity of long-term maintenance immunosuppression with medications that

Division of Nephrology and Hypertension, University of Miami Miller School of Medicine, 1120 NW 14th Street, Miami, FL 33136, USA
* Corresponding author. 1120 Northwest 14th Street, Room 813, Miami, FL 33136.
E-mail address: droth@med.miami.edu

Prim Care Clin Office Pract 41 (2014) 895–906
http://dx.doi.org/10.1016/j.pop.2014.08.009   **primarycare.theclinics.com**

present a host of adverse reactions and drug–drug interactions. With more than 17,000 kidney transplants being performed annually in the United States and almost 200,000 recipients alive with a functioning graft, it is not uncommon for PCPs to have several KTRs in their practice. The purpose of this review is to highlight medical management issues of practical usefulness to the PCP who is involved in the care of KTRs.

HYPERTENSION

Hypertension is often encountered in the management of KTRs with the prevalence reported to be from 50% to 90%.[1] Poorly controlled blood pressure has been shown to be an independent risk factor for cardiovascular disease (CVD) after kidney transplantation and is also associated with an increased risk of graft failure.[2–4] Studies in the general population have conclusively demonstrated that aggressive treatment of HTN is associated with a significant reduction in the incidence of cardiovascular events and a reduction in overall patient mortality.[5] These outcomes have been demonstrated in both observational and randomized clinical trials and although similar trials have not been performed in the transplant population, these results have been extrapolated to apply to the KTR as well.

The goals for treatment of HTN in the KTR have been mostly adopted from guidelines directed to the care of the general population. This includes reducing the systolic blood pressure to 140 mm Hg or less and diastolic blood pressure to 90 mm Hg or less for low-risk patients. In high-risk patients, such as those with diabetes mellitus (DM) or chronic kidney disease (CKD), the recommendation is to reduce the systolic blood pressure to 130 mm Hg or less and diastolic blood pressure to 80 mm Hg or less.[5,6]

The pathogenesis of HTN in the KTR shares many similar etiologies as in the general population; however, several other possibilities should also be considered. It has been clearly demonstrated that certain immunosuppressive medications can contribute to an increase in blood pressure or worsen blood pressure control. Calcineurin inhibitors (CNI) such as tacrolimus and cyclosporine are potent vasoconstrictors, and corticosteroids can be permissive of salt and water retention. Other clinical scenarios that might contribute to posttransplant HTN include acute and chronic allograft dysfunction and stenosis of the transplant renal artery. A careful assessment for each of these possibilities is part of the management of the KTR with poorly controlled or difficult to control blood pressure.

Treatment

It is generally accepted that all antihypertensive agents are useful in KTRs and the selection of the initial antihypertensive medication may be determined by factors such as race, the presence of comorbidities, and/or posttransplant complications (**Fig. 1**).

Calcium channel blockers are the most commonly prescribed antihypertensive for the KTR. The dihydropyridines, by virtue of their direct vasodilating properties, are a popular choice because they counteract the vasoconstrictive properties of the CNIs. Nondihydropyridine calcium channel blockers, such as verapamil and diltiazem, are less commonly used and should be avoided if at all possible because of their known inhibition of CYP3A with consequent increase in CNI blood levels.[7] Careful monitoring of CNI blood levels is warranted if calcium channel blockers, especially nondihydropyridines, are used.

β-Blockers are particularly useful in cases in which comorbidities such as congestive heart failure or coronary artery disease are present. The benefit of this class of antihypertensive on cardiac outcomes has been unequivocally demonstrated in the

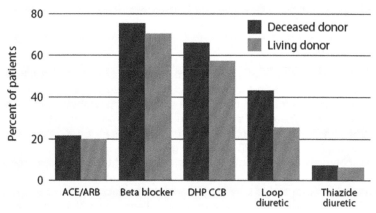

Fig. 1. Cardiovascular medication use in the first 6 months posttransplant. ACE, angiotensin-converting enzyme; ARB, angiotensin receptor blocker; CCB, calcium channel blocker; DHP, dihydropyridine. (*From* 2013 USRDS annual data report: atlas of chronic kidney disease and end-stage renal disease in the United States. Am J Kidney Dis 2014;63(2):e283–94.)

general population, and recent studies in KTRs share these favorable outcomes.[8,9] Possible adverse events associated with the use of β-blockers in KTRs include hyperkalemia, worsening dyslipidemia, and glucose intolerance. Most KTRs usually have CKD by GFR range and as a result often require a diuretic as part of the regimen to control their blood pressure. Thiazide diuretics are a good choice in patients with better levels of kidney function (ie, CKD 3a, 2, and 1) for controlling volume status in addition to increasing kaliuresis in patients predisposed to CNI-induced hyperkalemia. As a consequence of their adverse effect on glucose and lipid metabolism, the thiazides should be used cautiously in patients receiving CNIs (which can cause worsened glucose metabolism) and rapamycin, an immunosuppressive agent that can adversely affect lipid metabolism. Loop diuretics often become necessary in patients with more advanced stages of CKD. The indications for their use are similar to those of the thiazides; however, more careful monitoring of serum electrolytes and kidney function is necessary, especially early on after initiating treatment.

The beneficial effects of angiotensin-converting enzyme inhibitors (ACEI) and angiotensin receptor blockers on proteinuria and progression of kidney disease have been unequivocally demonstrated in both diabetic and nondiabetic disease of the native kidneys.[6] Of note, these agents have also been shown to be of benefit in KTRs, in whom their use was associated with a renal protective effect[10–12] and a survival advantage independent of the concomitant use of β-blockers.[8] For many years the ACEIs and angiotensin receptor blockers were not part of the HTN management protocols for KTRs out of a concern for worsening kidney function in a patient with a single kidney. Recent data have demonstrated that these agents can be used safely in the KTR and their use is clearly not contraindicated in the setting of kidney transplantation. In fact, these agents should be an integral part of the strategy to control proteinuria and slow the progression of CKD of the allograft. The only caveat is that they are usually avoided in the first 3 to 6 months posttransplantation, a period when even a small increase in the serum creatinine could be concerning and lead to extensive additional testing. ACEIs have been associated with the development of anemia in the KTR.[13] This adverse effect has been used to an advantage in the treatment of posttransplant erythrocytosis and ACEIs are the recommended treatment for this complication posttransplantation. Other concerns associated with the use of ACEIs and angiotensin receptor blockers are hyperkalemia and reduced renal perfusion, requiring that their use be carefully monitored in the KTR.[14,15]

DIABETES MELLITUS

DM has been identified as among the most important causes of morbidity and mortality among KTRs. Kidney recipients with DM can be divided into those patients whose diabetes predated the transplant and those who develop new-onset diabetes after transplant (NODAT). The definition of DM in KTRs follows the same criteria set by the World Health Organization and the American Diabetes Association, namely a fasting plasma glucose level of 126 mg/dL or greater (7.0 mmol/L), and/or a random plasma glucose level of 200 mg/dL or greater (11.1 mmol/L) plus the presence of symptoms and/or a 2-hour plasma glucose level of 200 mg/dL or greater (11.1 mmol/L), after an oral load of 75 g of anhydrous glucose.

NODAT is diagnosed in up to 42% of adult patients within the first 3 years after transplant (**Fig. 2**).[16] This high incidence is attributed to a number of known risk factors, such as positive family history, history of impaired glucose tolerance, Hispanic ethnicity, obesity, male gender, the use of corticosteroids, and the use of certain anti-rejection medications such as CNIs and sirolimus. In this subgroup of KTRs, the traditional complications of DM develop rapidly, including the risk of developing and/or accelerating the decline in allograft function and the known increased risk for unfavorable cardiovascular outcomes.

Current immunosuppressive protocols for KTRs rely heavily on the use of agents that have been identified to be diabetogenic, such as corticosteroids, CNIs, and mammalian target of rapamycin inhibitors such as rapamycin. The pathogenesis of CNI-induced NODAT is likely through several different mechanisms, including direct toxicity to the pancreatic β-cell[17] and inhibition of the transcription of the human insulin gene.[18] These effects are more pronounced in individuals with known concomitant risk factors and the simultaneous use of corticosteroids, especially when used at higher doses. Sirolimus has also been implicated in the development of NODAT.[19] Although the mechanism(s) have not yet been completely understood, chronic

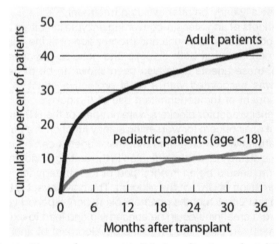

Fig. 2. Cumulative incidence of new-onset diabetes after transplant (NODAT) over time. (*From* 2013 USRDS annual data report: atlas of chronic kidney disease and end-stage renal disease in the United States. Am J Kidney Dis 2014;63(2):e283–94.)

mammalian target of rapamycin inhibition seems to increase peripheral insulin resistance.[20]

Treatment

The management of the KTR with glucose intolerance, whether it is preexisting DM or NODAT, can be challenging and is best accomplished through an active collaboration between the PCP, transplant center, endocrinologist, and dietician. The specific therapeutic goals of diabetic management in the KTR have not been defined; however, evidence from the general population suggests that a target hemoglobin A1C of less than 6.0% seems to be associated with an increased risk of mortality.[21] If the patient has not attained the target goal after all nonpharmacologic interventions have been implemented, the next step would be to add specific medications to the regimen (**Fig. 3**).

The appropriate choice of pharmacologic agent should take into account clinical issues unique to the patient, the desired level of glucose control, and the individual profile of the medications intended for use. Of note, an important factor in this decision process is the level of kidney function. As indicated, the majority of KTRs with a well-functioning allograft have some degree of CKD; thus, the choice of medication and dosing must take this into account. First-generation sulfonylureas such as chlorpropamide, tolazamide, and tolbutamide have been widely used in the past, but more recently they have fallen out of favor owing to their frequent interactions with the CNIs (increased blood levels).[22] Furthermore, their dose must be adjusted according to the level of GFR. Second-generation sulfonylureas are generally well tolerated with no need for dose adjustment for renal function, except for glyburide, which should be avoided in patients with a glomerular filtration rate (GFR) of less than 50 mL/min/1.73 m².[23] Caution with their use also includes more frequent monitoring of cyclosporine blood levels, because there can be an interaction with CNI metabolism.

The level of kidney function dictates the use of biguanides such as metformin and this agent is generally not used if the creatinine is 1.5 mg/dL or higher in men and 1.4 mg/dL or higher in women. Metformin is often recommended for obese patients with normal or near normal GFR. Most experts agree that phenformin is contraindicated in KTRs.

Thiazolidinediones (pioglitazone, rosiglitazone) do not require adjustment of dose for kidney function and there are no apparent pharmacologic interactions with the

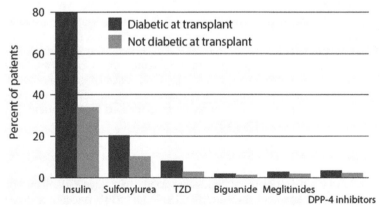

Fig. 3. Medications for diabetes control in the first 6 months posttransplant. TZD, thiazolidinedione. (*From* 2013 USRDS annual data report: atlas of chronic kidney disease and endstage renal disease in the United States. Am J Kidney Dis 2014;63(2):e283–94.)

most frequently used immunosuppressants (**Table 1**). Owing to their known capacity to cause fluid retention, they should be avoided in patients with acute kidney injury, advanced CKD, or congestive heart failure.

Meglitinides (repaglinide, nateglinide) are used commonly in the posttransplant patient with glucose intolerance. Recommended initial dosing is lower in patients with a GFR less than 40 mL/min/1.73 m^2 and uptitration of the dose should be done slowly based on patient tolerance. This class of diabetic medication is known to increase the blood levels of cyclosporine and therefore caution should be used, especially when using repaglinide.[24]

The incretin mimetic exenatide is only recommended for patients with GFR of 30 mL/min/1.73 m^2 or lower. It can be used concomitantly with the agents used in most current immunosuppressive protocols. Of note, the extended-release form carries a black box warning for patients with a personal or family history of medullary thyroid cancer and multiple endocrine neoplasia type 2.

The dipeptidyl peptidase 4 inhibitors such as vildagliptin should be avoided in patients receiving renal replacement therapy. They can be safely used for those patients with near normal GFR, but require careful adjustment of their dose in a step-wise fashion once the GFR falls below 50 mL/min/1.73 m^2. In addition, sitagliptin requires careful dosing when used in advanced CKD and end-stage renal disease.

Amylin analogs such as pramlintide require dosing adjustment for a GFR of 20 mL/min/1.73 m^2 or less and no major interactions have been documented with current immunosuppressive protocols.

α-Glucosidase inhibitors (acarbose, miglitol) should be avoided in patients whose kidney function is significantly reduced (GFR ≤ 25 mL/min/1.73 m^2). Acarbose is contraindicated in patients with a serum creatinine of 2 mg/dL or less (irrespective of gender) and miglitol should not be used in KTRs with a GRF of 25 mL/min/1.73 m^2 or less.

Insulin is frequently necessary for the successful management of KTRs with DM and NODAT. Insulin may be required in the immediate posttransplant period to control corticosteroid-induced hyperglycemia as well as to prevent acute diabetic complications, such as hyperosmolar state and ketoacidosis in patients with preexisting diabetes while receiving induction immunosuppression. Up to 80% of diabetics and nearly 35% of nondiabetic patients require insulin in the first 6 months posttransplantation.[16] For the long-term management of the KTR, insulin often assumes a central role in the treatment strategy, especially in patients with difficult-to-control diabetes and type 1 diabetics.

At present, there are limited clinical data to determine the ideal target hemoglobin A1c to prevent adverse cardiovascular outcomes in KTRs with DM or NODAT. All of the existing recommendations for the KTR have been extrapolated from large, controlled trials performed in the general population and suggest that intensive-glucose control (hemoglobin A1c ≤6%) in type 2 diabetics is associated with an increase in cardiovascular mortality.[21] In the absence of appropriate studies in the KTR population, it seems prudent to apply these guidelines to the diabetic patient in the post kidney transplant period as well.

DYSLIPIDEMIAS

Abnormalities in the metabolism of circulating lipoproteins (dyslipidemias) present a common clinical management issue in the KTR. In fact, CKD patients and KTRs are considered to be at the greatest risk for the development of CVD and have been shown to have some of the worst clinical outcomes.[25] Data obtained from the general population has demonstrated that significant reduction in the levels of low-density

Table 1
Common immunosuppressants: Common interactions and side effects

Agent	Classification/ Metabolism	Major Interactions	Side Effects
Tacrolimus, cyclosporine	Calcineurin inhibitors, cytochrome P-450	Decrease blood levels *Anti-TB drugs:* Rifampin, rifabutin, oxcarbazepine. *Anticonvulsants:* Barbiturates, phenytoin, carbamazepine *Antifungals:* Ketoconazole, fluconazole, itraconazole, voriconazole *Other:* St. John's Wort, ticlopidine, cholestiramine Increase blood levels *CCB:* Verapamil, diltiazem, amlodipine, nicardipine. *Antibiotics:* Erythromycin, clarithromycin. *Antiretrovirals:* Ritonavir. *Histamine blockers:* Cimetidine, ranitidine *Hormones:* Oral contraceptives, anabolic steroids, testosterone analogs, danazol. *Other:* Amiodarone, carvedilol, allopurinol, bromocriptine, grapefruit juice.	Nephrotoxicity Thrombotic Microangiopathy Vasoconstriction Hypertension Sodium retention Hyperkalemia Hypomagnesemia Hyperuricemia Hyperlipidemia New-onset DM Hair loss Gingival hyperplasia
Mycophenolate mofetil, (MMF), mycophenolic acid, (MPA)	Antimetabolites	Major interactions: Azathioprine (hematologic toxicity) Hydrxychloroquine (hematologic) Amoxicillin (increase level) Antacids, cholestyramine, sevelamer, (reduced absorption) Acyclovir, gancyclovir, (hematologic)	Diarrhea, (30%) Nausea, vomiting Leukopenia Congenital malformations Progressive multifocal leukoencephalopathy
Sirolimus, everolimus	mTOR inhibitors	Contraindicated Ketoconazole, mifepristone, voriconazole Similar interactions as CNIs because they share the same hepatic metabolic system	Potentiation of CNIs nephrotoxic effects De novo proteinuria Impaired hearing Impaired healing Embryotoxicity Fetotoxicity Hyperlipidemia Interstitial pneumonia

Abbreviations: CCB, calcium channel blockers; CNI, calcineurin inhibitor; DM, diabetes mellitus; mTOR, mammalian target of rapamycin; TB, tuberculosis.
From Danovitch G. Handbook of kidney transplantation. 5th edition. Philadelphia: Lippincott, Williams & Wilkins; 2010.

lipoprotein cholesterol (LDL-C) has a favorable impact on the risk of CVD.[26,27] This observation has also been confirmed in KTRs in whom the use of 3-hydroxy-3-meth-ylglutaryl coenzyme A (HMG-CoA) reductase inhibitors (statins) was linked to a reduction in adverse cardiovascular outcomes.[28,29] Increased levels of total cholesterol and LDL-C are particularly common in the KTR population and current guidelines recommend intensified screening protocols compared with the general population, initially during the first 3 months after transplantation and then at intervals that are appropriate to the specific case.[28]

KTRs are particularly at risk to develop secondary dyslipidemia associated with the presence of comorbid conditions such as diabetes and the nephrotic syndrome[30–32] (increase of total cholesterol, LDL-C cholesterol, triglycerides, or a combination) and should be instructed on appropriate dietary restrictions and to increase their level of physical activity when no contraindications are present, as well as the cessation of alcohol and tobacco use.

Of note, all efforts should be made to minimize the impact of correctable causes of dyslipidemia. For example, patients with the nephrotic syndrome often improve their levels of total cholesterol and LDL-C with reduction in proteinuria. The same consideration applies to metabolic conditions, such as diabetes. For those patients who develop severe dyslipidemia associated with the use of a medication such as rapamycin, consideration must be given to transitioning the patient to another immunosuppressant if this can be done safely. If the patient remains above goal after all steps have been implemented, the addition of pharmacologic agents is warranted.

The treatment of dyslipidemias in KTRs relies on the use of different classes of medications including the statins, fibrates, and ezetimibe (**Fig. 4**). The use of fibrates (fenofibrate) is reserved for those KTRs with markedly elevated serum triglycerides (triglycerides ≥500 mg/dL) in whom the concern for the development of pancreatitis takes precedence over the management of LDL-C.[28]

The management of the KTR with elevated LDL-C should rely on the use of statins. In fact, the most recent guidelines recommend the use of these agents in all KTRs, based on evidence showing that the 10-year risk for coronary death or nonfatal myocardial infarction is approximately 21.5%.[33] The ALERT trial (Assessment of

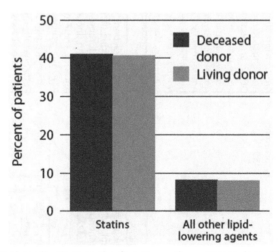

Fig. 4. Lipid control medications in the first 6 months posttransplant. (*From* 2013 USRDS annual data report: atlas of chronic kidney disease and end-stage renal disease in the United States. Am J Kidney Dis 2014;63(2):e283–94.)

Lescol in Renal Transplantation) demonstrated that fluvastatin (40–80 mg/d) was associated with a net reduction of 35% in the risk of cardiac death or nonfatal myocardial infarction, seemingly confirming results seen in studies of the general population.[29] The known risk burden for cardiovascular outcomes in KTRs emphasizes the need to achieve LDL-C levels below 100 mg/dL with an even more aggressive goal of 70 mg/dL or less in patients with known vascular disease.[28,33]

OBESITY

Obesity is a global health issue of major concern that has affected the end-stage renal disease population as well. Evidence obtained from observational studies in the general population suggests that obesity is an independent risk factor for CVD[34,35] as well as an important contributing factor to other chronic conditions such as HTN, DM, and dyslipidemia.[34,35] Although the evidence supporting these findings in KTRs has been obtained mostly from observational studies, there is a consensus opinion that the association of obesity with poor CVD outcomes extend to the KTR population as well.[36]

Treatment

Management of obesity in KTRs has been largely adopted from the experience obtained in the general population and includes a combination of diet, exercise, medications, and/or bariatric surgery. In general, all obese patients, regardless of the population group should be counseled to implement therapeutic life style changes, including diet and increased physical activity. The benefits of dieting in the general population have been demonstrated in several controlled trials[36] in which significant dietary modification has been able to achieve modest reductions in weight. In KTRs, dieting has been shown to be safe regardless of the specific diet,[37] especially when combined with increased physical activity.

The proper place for pharmacologic interventions in weight loss programs has remained controversial.[38] These agents have not been rigorously studied in the KTR population and any recommendations on their use are largely drawn from observational studies and case reports. Orlistat, for example, has been associated with interference in the intestinal absorption of cyclosporine.[36,39] Sibutramine can increase blood pressure and heart rate, and has not been studied in KTRs.[36] Rimonabant, which was never approved to use in the United States, was recently withdrawn from European markets owing to potentially serious side effects.

Bariatric surgical procedures can have a role in the management of obesity in the end-stage renal disease and kidney transplant population. Regardless of the specific procedure offered (gastric bypass, gastric banding, gastric sleeve), the effects on weight reduction can be significant and long-term weight losses of 25% or more from the baseline have been observed.[36,40]

SUMMARY

KTRs are a challenging group of patients to medically manage. The unique combination of multiple metabolic conditions, CKD, and the requirement for long-term maintenance immunosuppression place this cohort of patients at a significantly increased risk for cardiovascular morbidity and mortality. Successful management of this rapidly increasing population of patients requires a seamless collaboration between the PCP and the transplant center. Aggressive modification of cardiac risk factors coupled with effective management of CKD comorbidities and maintenance immunosuppression represent the key to long-term success.

REFERENCES

1. Ojo AO. Cardiovascular complications after renal transplantation and their prevention. Transplantation 2006;82:603–11.
2. Kasiske BL, Chakkera HA, Roel J. Explained and unexplained ischemic heart disease risk after renal transplantation. J Am Soc Nephrol 2000;11:1735–43.
3. Opelz G, Wujciak T, Ritz E. Association of chronic kidney graft failure with recipient blood pressure. Collaborative transplant study. Kidney Int 1998;53:217–22.
4. Mange KC, Feldman HI, Joffe MM, et al. Blood pressure and the survival of renal allografts from living donors. J Am Soc Nephrol 2004;15:187–93.
5. Chobanian AV, Bakris GL, Black HR, et al. The seventh report of the Joint National Committee on prevention, detection, evaluation and treatment of high blood pressure: the JNC 7 report. JAMA 2003;289:2560–72.
6. Kidney Disease Outcomes Quality Initiative (K/DOQI). K/DOQI clinical practice guidelines on hypertension and antihypertensive agents in chronic kidney disease. Am J Kidney Dis 2004;43:S1–290.
7. Danovitch G. Handbook of kidney transplantation. 5th edition. Philadelphia: Lippincott, Williams & Wilkins; 2010. p. 77–126.
8. Aftab W, Varadarajan P, Rasool S, et al. Beta and angiotensin blockades are associated with 10-year survival in renal transplant recipients. J Am Heart Assoc 2013;2:e000091. http://dx.doi.org/10.1161/JAHA.112.000091.
9. Curtis JJ, Luke RG, Jones P, et al. Hypertension in cyclosporine-treated renal transplant recipients is sodium dependent. Am J Med 1988;85:134–8.
10. Inigo P, Campistol JM, Saracho R, et al. Renoprotective effects of losartan in renal transplant recipients. Results of a retrospective study. Nephron Clin Pract 2003; 95:c84–90.
11. Artz MA, Hilbrands LB, Borm G, et al. Blockade of the renin-angiotensin system increases graft survival in patients with chronic allograft nephropathy. Nephrol Dial Transplant 2004;19:2852–7.
12. Suwelack B, Kobelt V, Erfmann M, et al. Long-term follow-up of ACE-inhibitor versus beta-blocker treatment and their effects on blood pressure and kidney function in renal transplant recipients. Transpl Int 2003;16:313–20.
13. Demetrios V, Vlahakos MD, Vincent J, et al. Enalapril-associated anemia in renal transplant recipients treated for hypertension. Am J Kidney Dis 1991;17(2): 199–205.
14. Stigant CE, Cohen J, Vivera M, et al. ACE inhibitors and angiotensin II antagonists in renal transplantation: an analysis of safety and efficacy. Am J Kidney Dis 2000; 35:58–63.
15. American Diabetes Association. Diagnosis and classification of diabetes mellitus. Diabetes Care 2009;32(Suppl 1):S62–7.
16. 2013 USRDS annual data report: atlas of chronic kidney disease and end-stage renal disease in the United States. Am J Kidney Dis 2014;63(2):e283–94 Supplement.
17. Ajabnoor MA, El-Naggar MM, Elayat AA, et al. Functional and morphological study of cultured pancreatic islets treated with cyclosporine. Life Sci 2007;80: 345–55.
18. Oetjen E, Baun D, Beimesche S, et al. Inhibition of human insulin gene transcription by the immunosuppressive drugs cyclosporine A and tacrolimus in primary, mature islets of transgenic mice. Mol Pharmacol 2003;63:1289–95.
19. Johnston O, Rose CL, Webster AC, et al. Sirolimus is associated with new-onset diabetes in kidney transplant recipients. J Am Soc Nephrol 2008;19(7):1411–8.

20. Teutonico A, Schena PF, Di Paolo S. Glucose metabolism in renal transplant recipients: effect of calcineurin inhibitor withdrawal and conversion to sirolimus. J Am Soc Nephrol 2005;16:3128–35.
21. Gerstein HC, Miller ME, Byington RP, et al. Effects of intensive glucose lowering in type 2 diabetes. N Engl J Med 2008;358:2545–59.
22. Harrower AD. Pharmacokinetics of oral antihyperglycaemic agents in patients with renal insufficiency. Clin Pharmacokinet 1996;31:111–9.
23. Krepinsky J, Ingram AJ, Clase CM. Prolonged sulfonylurea-induced hypoglycemia in diabetic patients with end-stage renal disease. Am J Kidney Dis 2000; 35:500–5.
24. Kajosaari LI, Niemi M, Neuvonen M, et al. Cyclosporine markedly raises the plasma concentrations of repaglinide. Clin Pharmacol Ther 2005;78:388–99.
25. National Kidney Foundation. K/DOQI clinical practice guidelines for managing dyslipidemias in chronic kidney disease. Am J Kidney Dis 2003;41(Suppl 3): S1–91.
26. Sacks FM, Tonkin AM, Shepherd J, et al. Effect of pravastatin on coronary disease events in subgroups defined by coronary risk factors. The prospective pravastatin pooling project. Circulation 2000;102:1893–900.
27. Lewington S, Whitlock G, Clarke R, et al, Prospective Studies Collaboration. Blood cholesterol and vascular mortality by age, sex, and blood pressure: a meta-analysis of individual data from 61 prospective studies with 55,000 vascular deaths. Lancet 2007;370:1829–39.
28. Kasiske B, Cosio FG, Beto J, et al. Clinical practice guidelines for managing dyslipidemias in kidney transplant patients: a report from the Managing Dyslipidemias in Chronic Kidney Disease Work Group of the National Kidney Foundation Kidney Disease Outcomes Quality Initiative. Am J Transplant 2004;4(Suppl 7): 13–53.
29. Holdaas H, Fellström B, Jardine AG, et al, Assessment of LEscol in Renal Transplantation (ALERT) Study Investigators. Effect of fluvastatin on cardiac outcomes in renal transplant recipients: a multicentre, randomised, placebo-controlled trial. Lancet 2003;361:2024–31.
30. Verges BL. Dyslipidaemia in diabetes mellitus. Review of the main lipoprotein abnormalities and their consequences on the development of atherogenesis. Diabetes Metab 1999;25(Suppl 3):32–40.
31. Kaysen GA, Don B, Schambelan M. Proteinuria, albumin synthesis and hyperlipidemia in the nephrotic syndrome. Nephrol Dial Transplant 1991;6:141–9.
32. Hoogeveen RC, Ballantyne CM, Pownall HJ, et al. Effect of sirolimus on the metabolism of ApoB100-containing lipoproteins in renal transplant patients. Transplantation 2001;72:1244–50.
33. Tonelli M, Wanner C. Lipid management in chronic kidney disease: synopsis of the kidney disease: Improving Global Outcomes 2013 clinical practice guideline. Ann Intern Med 2014;160:182–9.
34. National Heart, Lung, and Blood Institute. The practical guide Identification, evaluation, and treatment of overweight and obesity in adults. Bethesda (MD): US Department of Health and Human Services Public Health Service; National Institutes of Health; 2000.
35. Eckel RH, Krauss RM. American Heart Association call to action: obesity as a major risk factor for coronary heart disease. AHA Nutrition Committee. Circulation 1998;97:2099–100.
36. National Kidney Foundation. KDIGO clinical practice guideline for the care of kidney transplant recipients. Am J Transplant 2009;9(Suppl 3):S71–9.

37. Patel MG. The effect of dietary intervention on weight gains after renal transplantation. J Ren Nutr 1998;8:137–41.
38. Li Z, Maglione M, Tu W, et al. Meta-analysis: pharmacologic treatment of obesity. Ann Intern Med 2005;142:532–46.
39. Barbaro D, Orsini P, Pallini S, et al. Obesity in transplant patients: case report showing interference of orlistat with absorption of cyclosporine and review of literature. Endocr Pract 2002;8:124–6.
40. Sjostrom L, Narbro K, Sjostrom CD, et al. Effects of bariatric surgery on mortality in Swedish obese subjects. N Engl J Med 2007;357:741–52.

Index

Note: Page numbers of article titles are in **boldface** type.

Prim Care Clin Office Pract 41 (2014) 907–920
http://dx.doi.org/10.1016/S0095-4543(14)00119-5
0095-4543/14/$ – see front matter © 2014 Elsevier Inc. All rights reserved.

primarycare.theclinics.com

United States Postal Service

Statement of Ownership, Management, and Circulation
(All Periodicals Publications Except Requestor Publications)

1. Publication Title	2. Publication Number		3. Filing Date
Primary Care: Clinics in Office Practice	0 4 4 - 6 9 0		9/14/14

4. Issue Frequency	5. Number of Issues Published Annually	6. Annual Subscription Price
Mar, Jun, Sep, Dec	4	$225.00

7. Complete Mailing Address of Known Office of Publication (*Not printer*) (*Street, city, county, state, and ZIP+4®*)

Elsevier Inc.
360 Park Avenue South
New York, NY 10010-1710

Contact Person
Stephen R. Bushing
Telephone (*Include area code*)
215-239-3688

8. Complete Mailing Address of Headquarters or General Business Office of Publisher (*Not printer*)

Elsevier Inc., 360 Park Avenue South, New York, NY 10010-1710

9. Full Names and Complete Mailing Addresses of Publisher, Editor, and Managing Editor (*Do not leave blank*)

Publisher (*Name and complete mailing address*)

Linda Belfus, Elsevier, Inc., 1600 John F. Kennedy Blvd. Suite 1800, Philadelphia, PA 19103-2899

Editor (*Name and complete mailing address*)

Jessica McCool, Elsevier, Inc., 1600 John F. Kennedy Blvd. Suite 1800, Philadelphia, PA 19103-2899

Managing Editor (*Name and complete mailing address*)

Adrianne Brigido, Elsevier, Inc., 1600 John F. Kennedy Blvd. Suite 1800, Philadelphia, PA 19103-2899

10. Owner (*Do not leave blank. If the publication is owned by a corporation, give the name and address of the corporation immediately followed by the names and addresses of all stockholders owning or holding 1 percent or more of the total amount of stock. If not owned by a corporation, give the names and addresses of the individual owners. If owned by a partnership or other unincorporated firm, give its name and address as well as those of each individual owner. If the publication is published by a nonprofit organization, give its name and address.*)

Full Name	Complete Mailing Address
Wholly owned subsidiary of	1600 John F. Kennedy Blvd, Ste. 1800
Reed/Elsevier, US holdings	Philadelphia, PA 19103-2899

11. Known Bondholders, Mortgagees, and Other Security Holders Owning or Holding 1 Percent or More of Total Amount of Bonds, Mortgages, or Other Securities. If none, check box ☐ None

Full Name	Complete Mailing Address
N/A	

12. Tax Status (*For completion by nonprofit organizations authorized to mail at nonprofit rates*) (*Check one*)
The purpose, function, and nonprofit status of this organization and the exempt status for federal income tax purposes:
☐ Has Not Changed During Preceding 12 Months
☐ Has Changed During Preceding 12 Months (*Publisher must submit explanation of change with this statement*)

PS Form 3526, August 2012 (Page 1 of 3 (Instructions Page 3)) PSN 7530-01-000-9931 PRIVACY NOTICE: See our Privacy policy in www.usps.com

---

13. Publication Title	14. Issue Date for Circulation Data Below
Primary Care: Clinics in Office Practice	September 2014

15. Extent and Nature of Circulation		Average No. Copies Each Issue During Preceding 12 Months	No. Copies of Single Issue Published Nearest to Filing Date
a. Total Number of Copies (*Net press run*)		246	216
b. Paid Circulation (By Mail and Outside the Mail)	(1) Mailed Outside-County Paid Subscriptions Stated on PS Form 3541. (*Include paid distribution above nominal rate, advertiser's proof copies, and exchange copies*)	148	136
	(2) Mailed In-County Paid Subscriptions Stated on PS Form 3541 (*Include paid distribution above nominal rate, advertiser's proof copies, and exchange copies*)		
	(3) Paid Distribution Outside the Mails Including Sales Through Dealers and Carriers, Street Vendors, Counter Sales, and Other Paid Distribution Outside USPS®	23	21
	(4) Paid Distribution by Other Classes Mailed Through the USPS (e.g. First-Class Mail®)		
c. Total Paid Distribution (*Sum of 15b (1), (2), (3), and (4)*)	▶	171	157
d. Free or Nominal Rate Distribution (By Mail and Outside the Mail)	(1) Free or Nominal Rate Outside-County Copies Included on PS Form 3541	29	34
	(2) Free or Nominal Rate In-County Copies Included on PS Form 3541		
	(3) Free or Nominal Rate Copies Mailed at Other Classes Through the USPS (e.g. First-Class Mail)		
	(4) Free or Nominal Rate Distribution Outside the Mail (Carriers or other means)		
e. Total Free or Nominal Rate Distribution (Sum of 15d (1), (2), (3) and (4)	▶	29	34
f. Total Distribution (Sum of 15c and 15e)	▶	200	191
g. Copies not Distributed (See instructions to publishers #4 (page #3))	▶	46	25
h. Total (Sum of 15f and g)	▶	246	216
i. Percent Paid (15c divided by 15f times 100)	▶	85.50%	82.20%

16. Total circulation includes electronic copies. Report circulation on PS Form 3526-X worksheet.

17. Publication of Statement of Ownership
If the publication is a general publication, publication of this statement is required. Will be printed in the December 2014 issue of this publication.

18. Signature and Title of Editor, Publisher, Business Manager, or Owner	Date
Stephen R. Bushing	September 14, 2014
Stephen R. Bushing – Inventory Distribution Coordinator	

I certify that all information furnished on this form is true and complete. I understand that anyone who furnishes false or misleading information on this form or who omits material or information requested on the form may be subject to criminal sanctions (including fines and imprisonment) and/or civil sanctions (including civil penalties).

PS Form 3526, August 2012 (Page 2 of 3)

Moving?

Make sure your subscription moves with you!

To notify us of your new address, find your **Clinics Account Number** (located on your mailing label above your name), and contact customer service at:

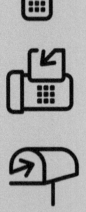

Email: journalscustomerservice-usa@elsevier.com

800-654-2452 (subscribers in the U.S. & Canada)
314-447-8871 (subscribers outside of the U.S. & Canada)

Fax number: 314-447-8029

Elsevier Health Sciences Division
Subscription Customer Service
3251 Riverport Lane
Maryland Heights, MO 63043

*To ensure uninterrupted delivery of your subscription, please notify us at least 4 weeks in advance of move.

Printed and bound by CPI Group (UK) Ltd, Croydon, CR0 4YY

03/10/2024

01040491-0001